1/12

PSYCHIATRIC
TALES

PSYCHIATRIC
TALES

ELEVEN GRAPHIC STORIES
ABOUT MENTAL ILLNESS

DARRYL CUNNINGHAM

BLOOMSBURY

New York   Berlin   London   Sydney

Published by Bloomsbury USA, New York

All papers used by Bloomsbury USA are natural, recyclable products made from wood
grown in well-managed forests. The manufacturing processes conform to the
environmental regulations of the country of origin.

LIBRARY OF CONGRESS CATALOGING—IN—PUBLICATION DATA HAS BEEN APPLIED FOR.

ISBN: 978-1-60819-278-6

First published in the United Kingdom in 2010 by Blank Slate Books Limited

First U.S. Edition 2011

1 3 5 7 9 10 8 6 4 2

Printed in the U.S.A. by Quad/Graphics, Fairfield, Pennsylvania

GRAPH CUNNINGHAM

INTRODUCTION

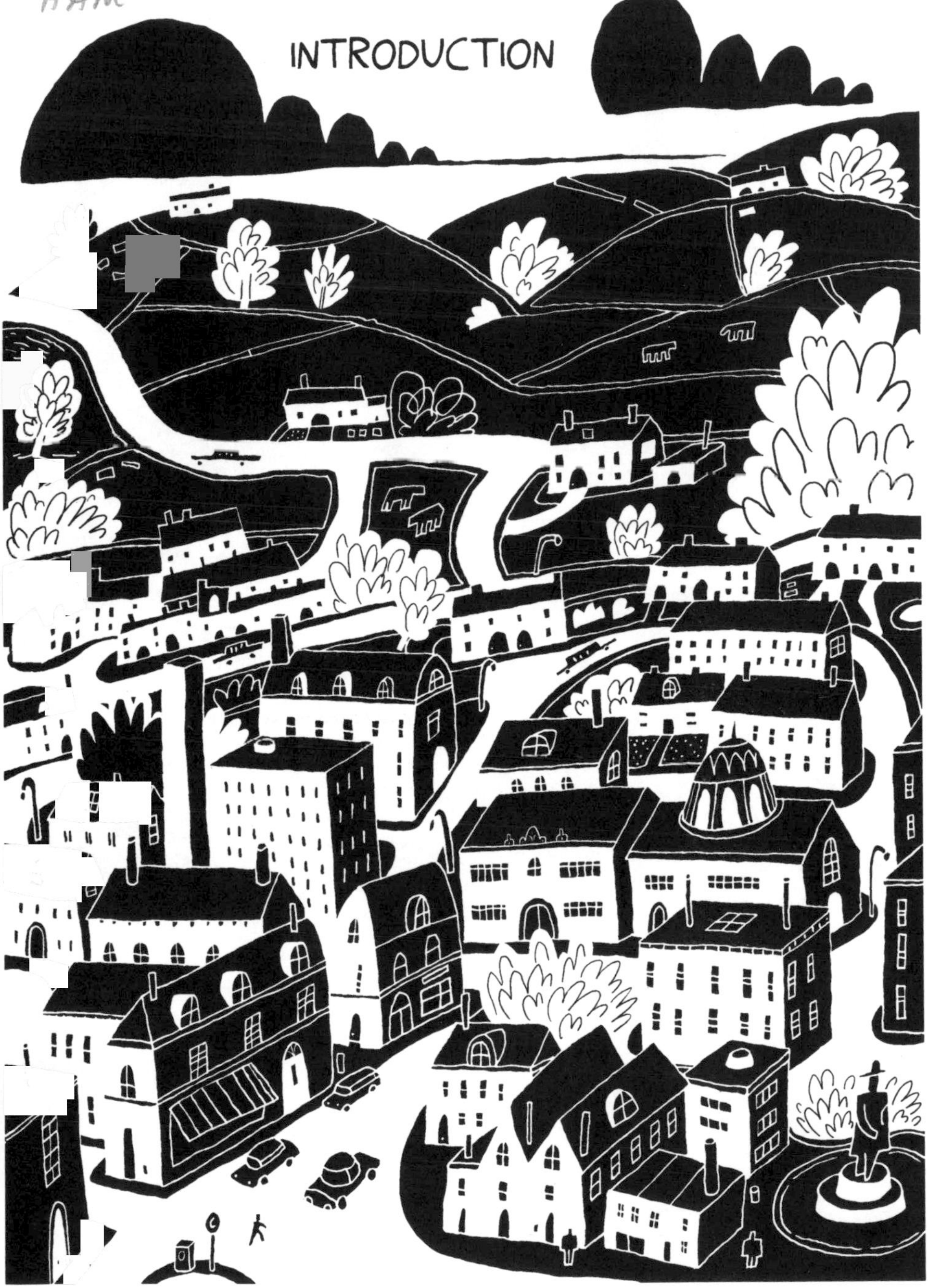

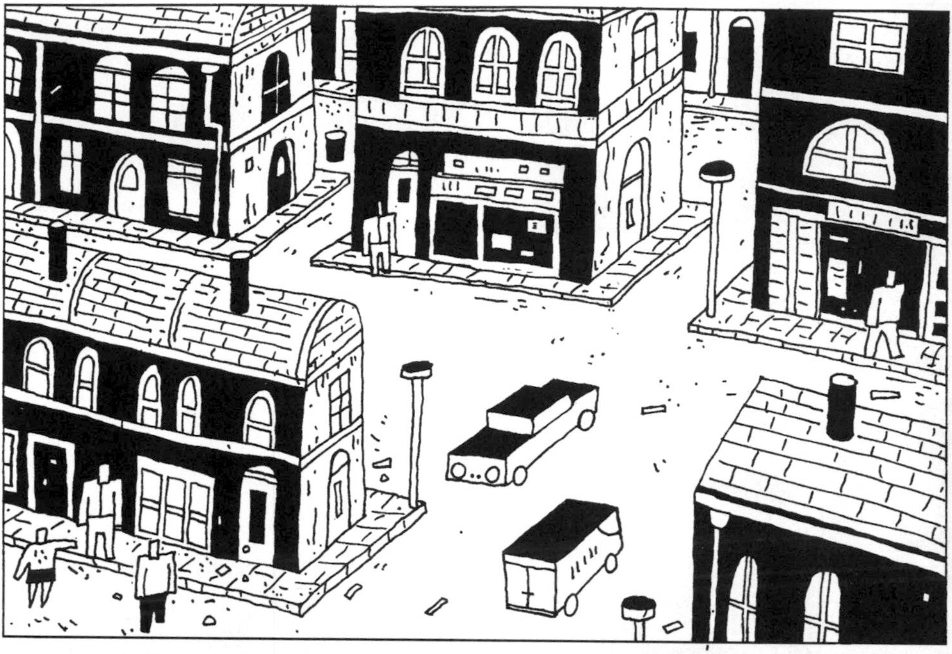

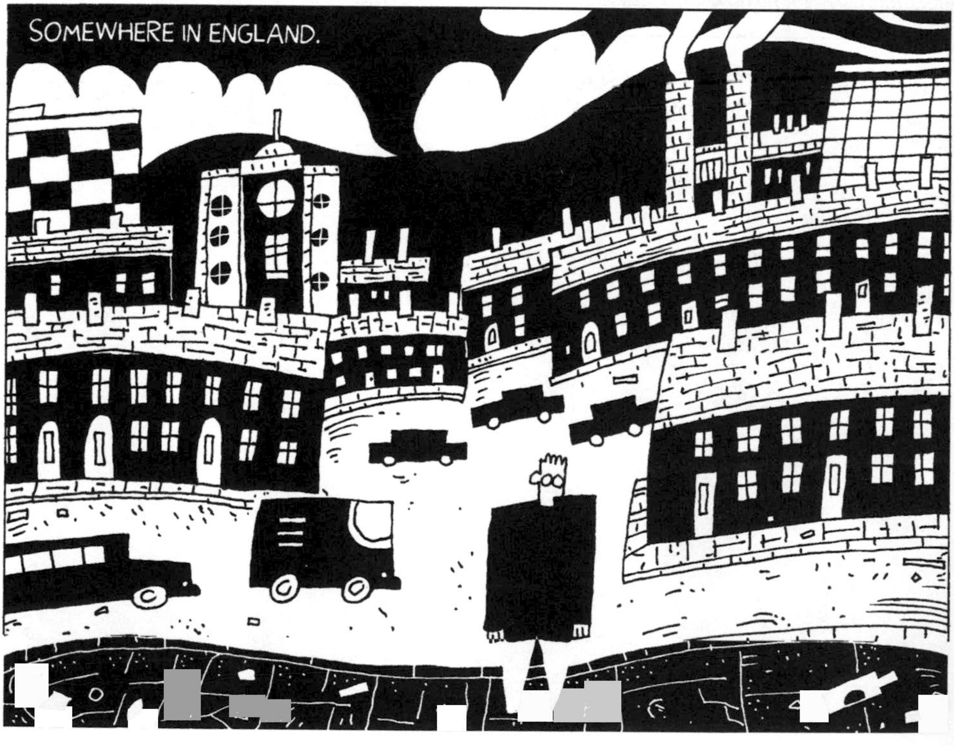
SOMEWHERE IN ENGLAND.

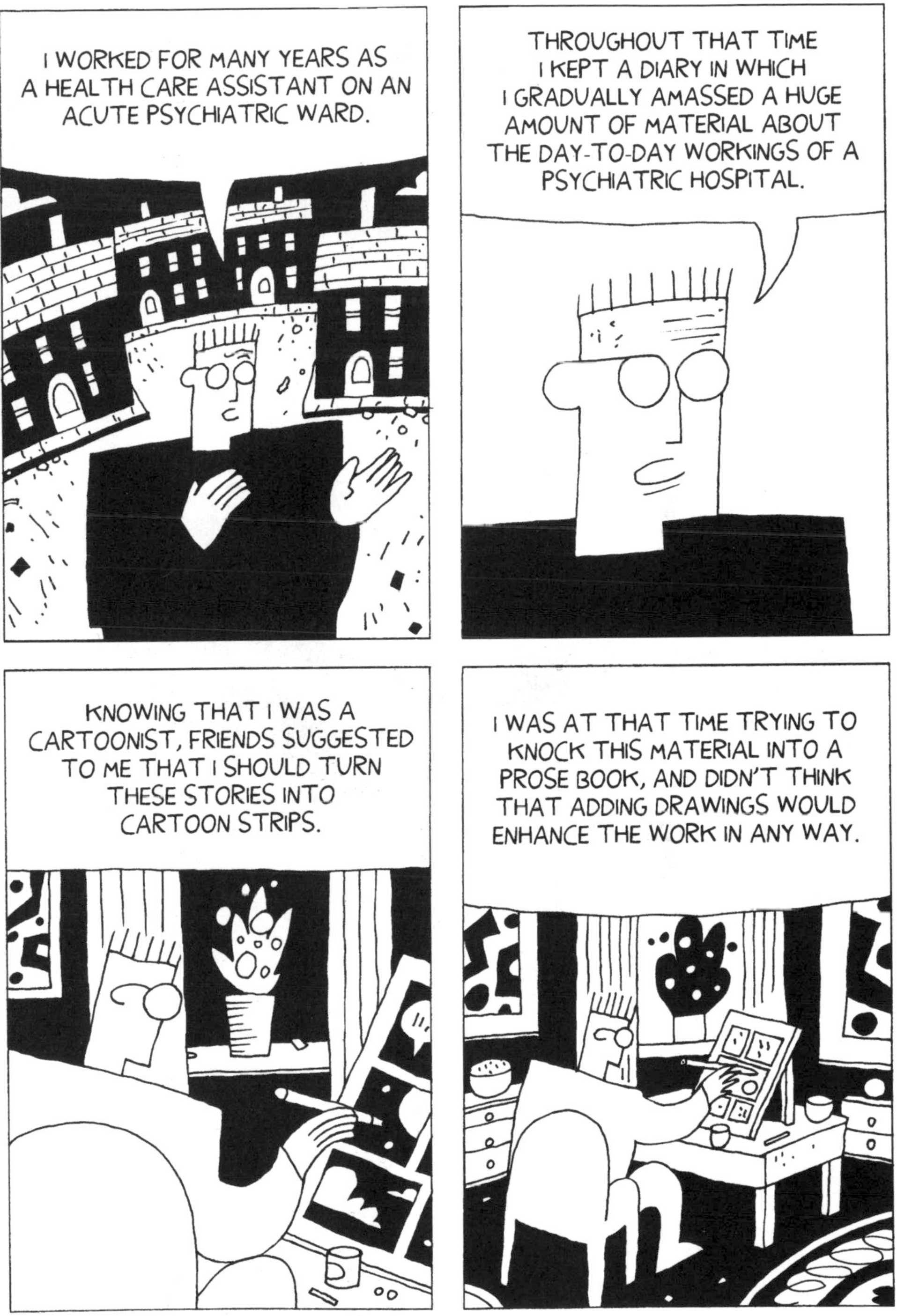
I WORKED FOR MANY YEARS AS A HEALTH CARE ASSISTANT ON AN ACUTE PSYCHIATRIC WARD.
THROUGHOUT THAT TIME I KEPT A DIARY IN WHICH I GRADUALLY AMASSED A HUGE AMOUNT OF MATERIAL ABOUT THE DAY-TO-DAY WORKINGS OF A PSYCHIATRIC HOSPITAL.
KNOWING THAT I WAS A CARTOONIST, FRIENDS SUGGESTED TO ME THAT I SHOULD TURN THESE STORIES INTO CARTOON STRIPS.
I WAS AT THAT TIME TRYING TO KNOCK THIS MATERIAL INTO A PROSE BOOK, AND DIDN'T THINK THAT ADDING DRAWINGS WOULD ENHANCE THE WORK IN ANY WAY.

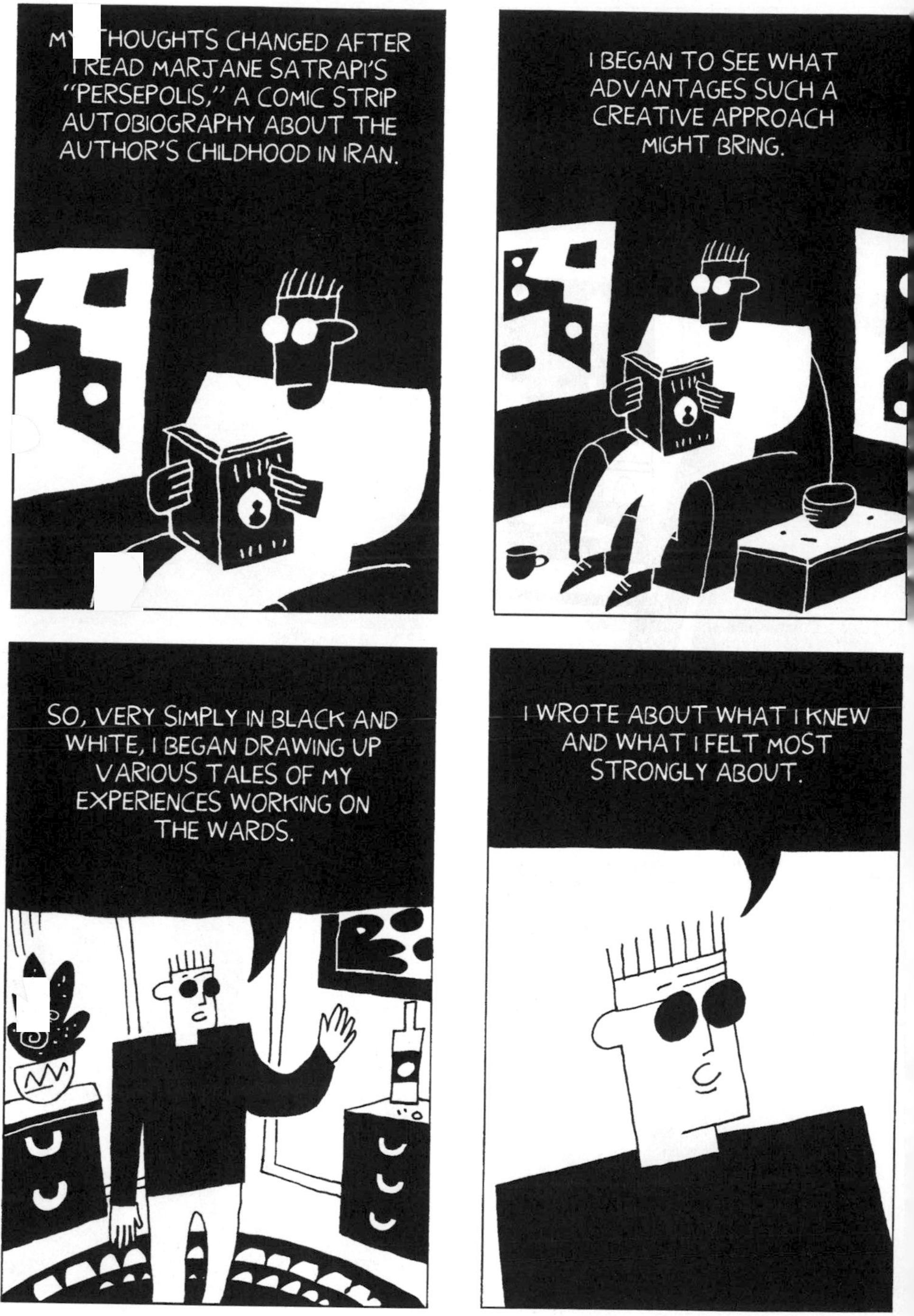
MY THOUGHTS CHANGED AFTER I READ MARJANE SATRAPI'S "PERSEPOLIS," A COMIC STRIP AUTOBIOGRAPHY ABOUT THE AUTHOR'S CHILDHOOD IN IRAN.
I BEGAN TO SEE WHAT ADVANTAGES SUCH A CREATIVE APPROACH MIGHT BRING.
SO, VERY SIMPLY IN BLACK AND WHITE, I BEGAN DRAWING UP VARIOUS TALES OF MY EXPERIENCES WORKING ON THE WARDS.
I WROTE ABOUT WHAT I KNEW AND WHAT I FELT MOST STRONGLY ABOUT.

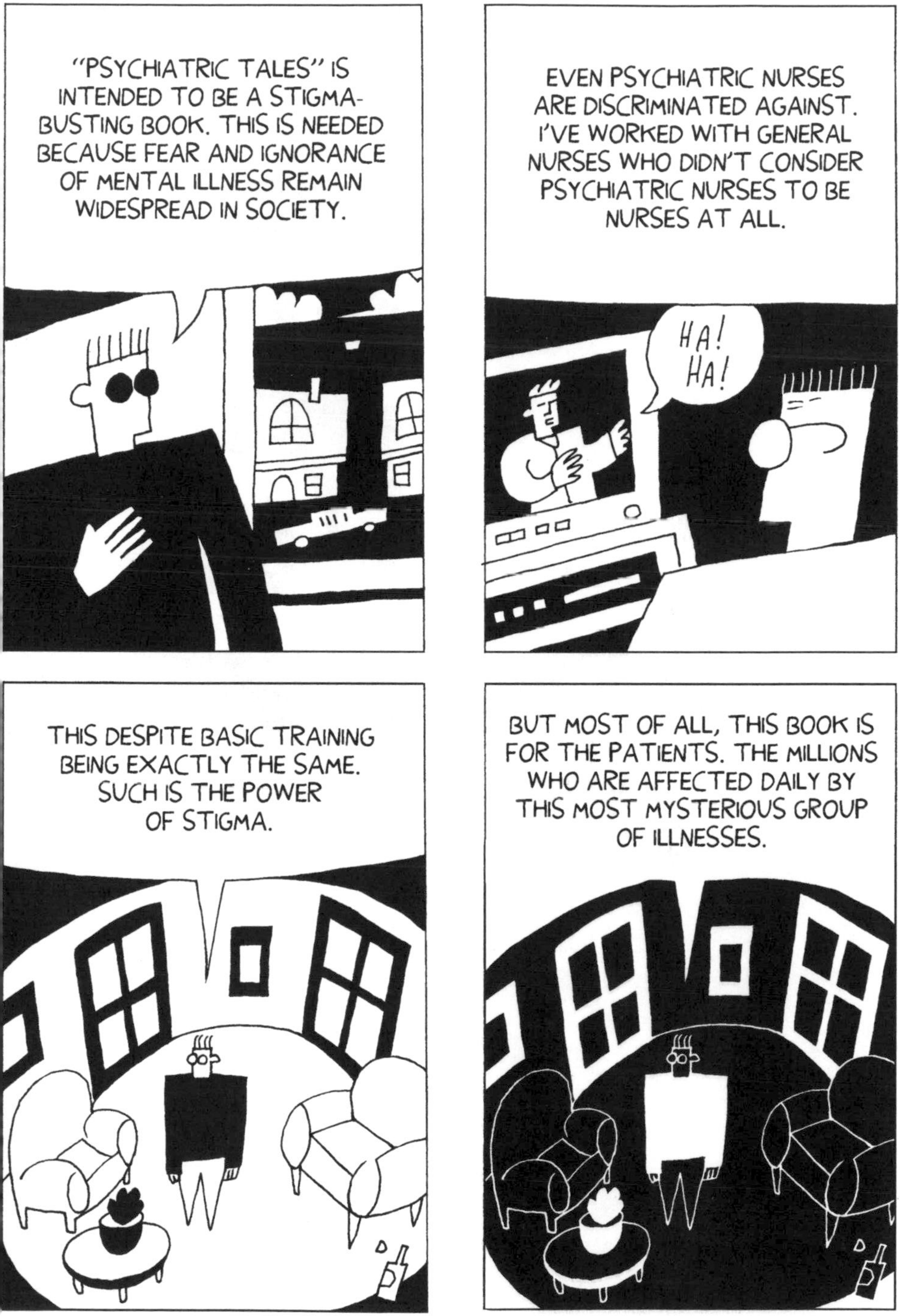
"PSYCHIATRIC TALES" IS INTENDED TO BE A STIGMA-BUSTING BOOK. THIS IS NEEDED BECAUSE FEAR AND IGNORANCE OF MENTAL ILLNESS REMAIN WIDESPREAD IN SOCIETY.
EVEN PSYCHIATRIC NURSES ARE DISCRIMINATED AGAINST. I'VE WORKED WITH GENERAL NURSES WHO DIDN'T CONSIDER PSYCHIATRIC NURSES TO BE NURSES AT ALL.
HA! HA!
THIS DESPITE BASIC TRAINING BEING EXACTLY THE SAME. SUCH IS THE POWER OF STIGMA.
BUT MOST OF ALL, THIS BOOK IS FOR THE PATIENTS. THE MILLIONS WHO ARE AFFECTED DAILY BY THIS MOST MYSTERIOUS GROUP OF ILLNESSES.

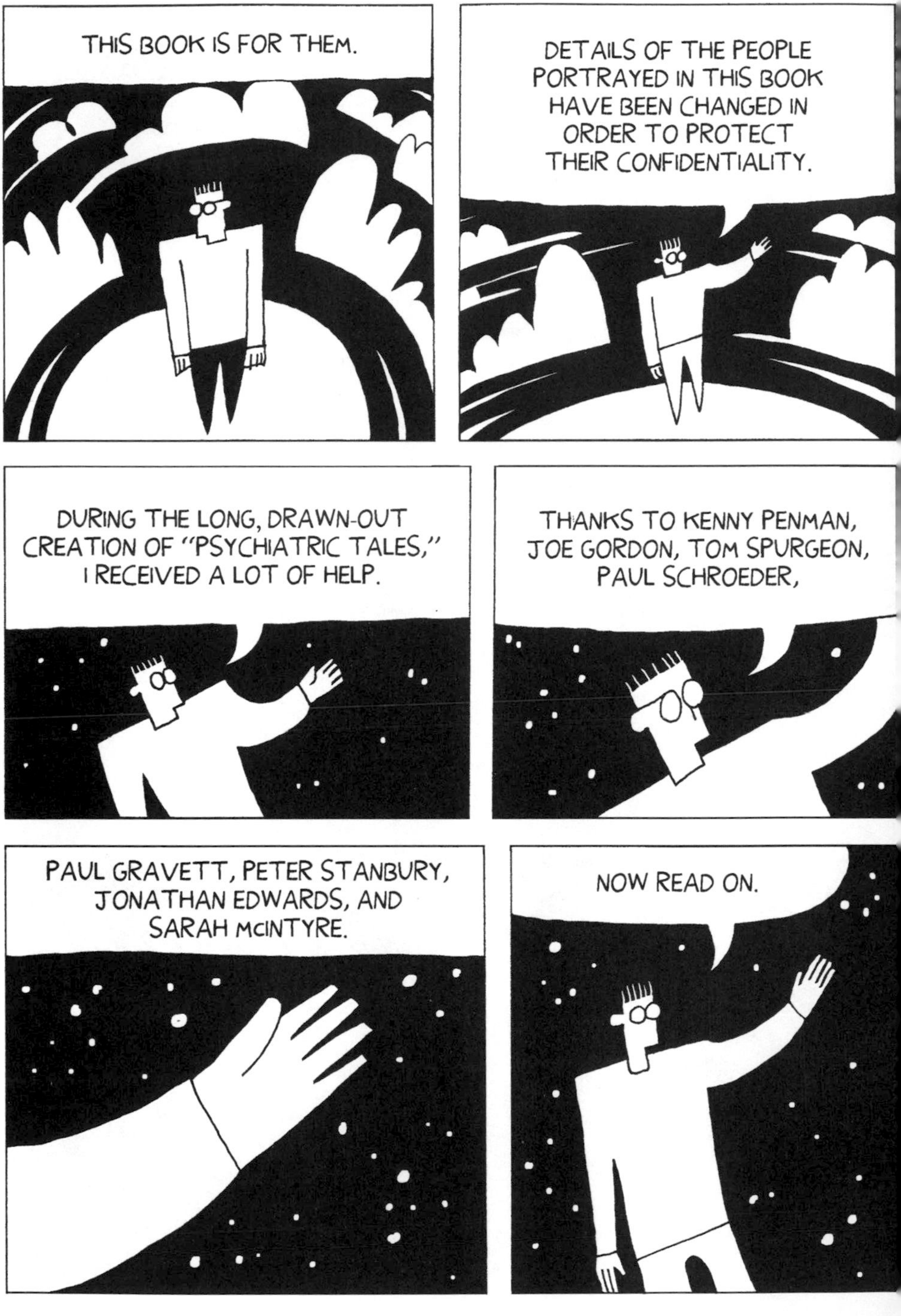
THIS BOOK IS FOR THEM.
DETAILS OF THE PEOPLE PORTRAYED IN THIS BOOK HAVE BEEN CHANGED IN ORDER TO PROTECT THEIR CONFIDENTIALITY.
DURING THE LONG, DRAWN-OUT CREATION OF "PSYCHIATRIC TALES," I RECEIVED A LOT OF HELP.
THANKS TO KENNY PENMAN, JOE GORDON, TOM SPURGEON, PAUL SCHROEDER,
PAUL GRAVETT, PETER STANBURY, JONATHAN EDWARDS, AND SARAH McINTYRE.
NOW READ ON.

PSYCHIATRIC
TALES

DEMENTIA
WARD

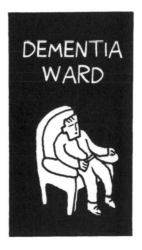

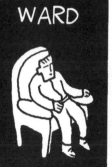

DEMENTIA WARD

ON THE DEMENTIA WARD PATIENTS ARE OFTEN UNAWARE THAT THEY'RE IN A HOSPITAL.

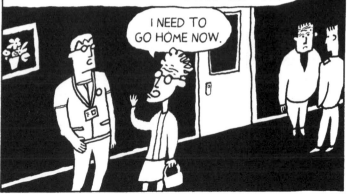

I NEED TO GO HOME NOW.

THE CAPACITY TO INTERPRET INFORMATION AND THEN RELATE THAT INFORMATION TO THE PRESENT MOMENT VANISHES ONCE DEMENTIA GETS A GRIP ON THE MIND.

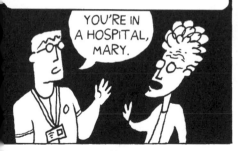

YOU'RE IN A HOSPITAL, MARY.

STAFF ON THE DEMENTIA WARD WEAR UNIFORMS, BUT EVEN THIS MAY NOT TIP THE PATIENTS OFF.

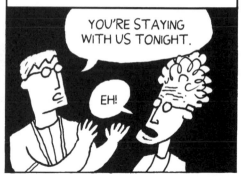

YOU'RE STAYING WITH US TONIGHT.

EH!

MANY WILL BELIEVE THAT THEY'RE STAYING IN A HOTEL FROM WHICH THEY'LL BE RETURNING HOME SOON.

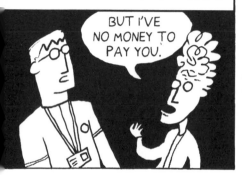

BUT I'VE NO MONEY TO PAY YOU.

DON'T WORRY ABOUT ALL THAT, MARY. IT'S ALL BEEN PAID FOR.

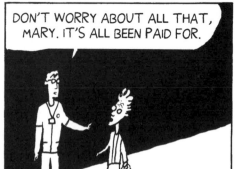

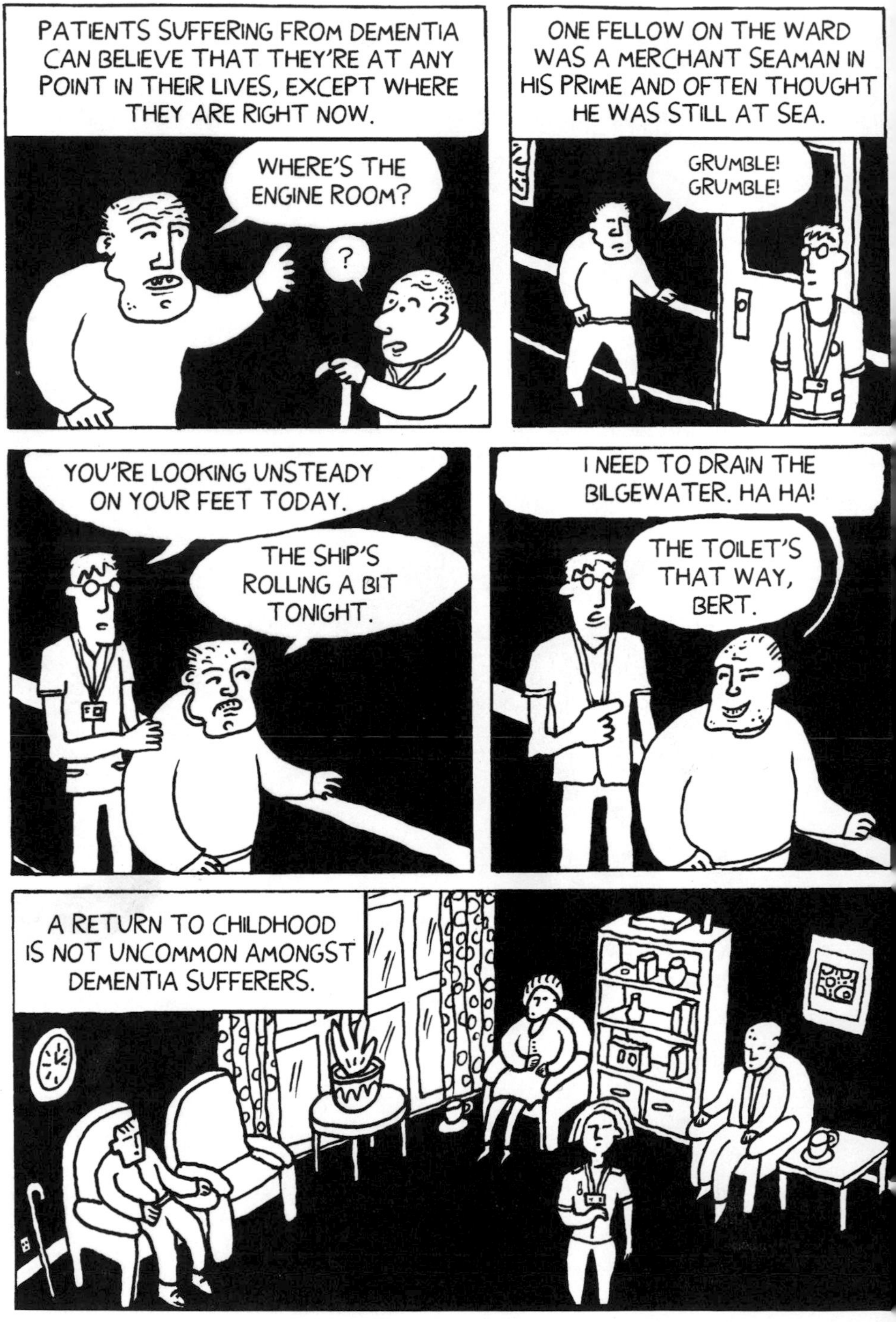
PATIENTS SUFFERING FROM DEMENTIA CAN BELIEVE THAT THEY'RE AT ANY POINT IN THEIR LIVES, EXCEPT WHERE THEY ARE RIGHT NOW.
WHERE'S THE ENGINE ROOM?
?
ONE FELLOW ON THE WARD WAS A MERCHANT SEAMAN IN HIS PRIME AND OFTEN THOUGHT HE WAS STILL AT SEA.
GRUMBLE! GRUMBLE!
YOU'RE LOOKING UNSTEADY ON YOUR FEET TODAY.
THE SHIP'S ROLLING A BIT TONIGHT.
I NEED TO DRAIN THE BILGEWATER. HA HA!
THE TOILET'S THAT WAY, BERT.
A RETURN TO CHILDHOOD IS NOT UNCOMMON AMONGST DEMENTIA SUFFERERS.

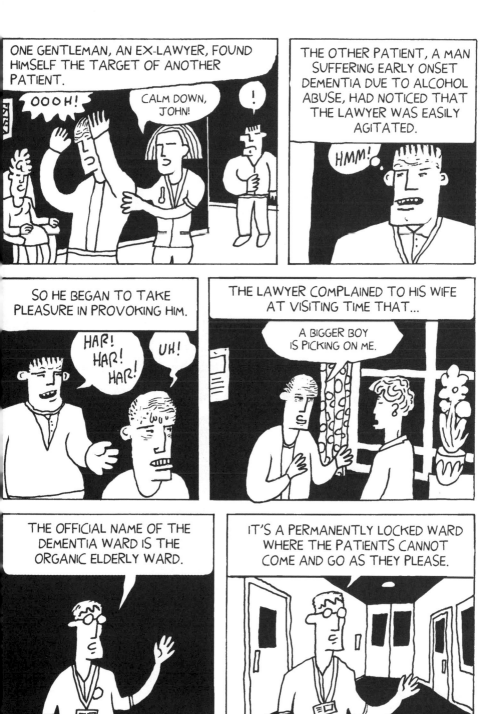

ONE GENTLEMAN, AN EX-LAWYER, FOUND HIMSELF THE TARGET OF ANOTHER PATIENT.

OOOH!

CALM DOWN, JOHN!

!

THE OTHER PATIENT, A MAN SUFFERING EARLY ONSET DEMENTIA DUE TO ALCOHOL ABUSE, HAD NOTICED THAT THE LAWYER WAS EASILY AGITATED.

HMM!

SO HE BEGAN TO TAKE PLEASURE IN PROVOKING HIM.

HAR! HAR! HAR!

UH!

THE LAWYER COMPLAINED TO HIS WIFE AT VISITING TIME THAT...

A BIGGER BOY IS PICKING ON ME.

THE OFFICIAL NAME OF THE DEMENTIA WARD IS THE ORGANIC ELDERLY WARD.

IT'S A PERMANENTLY LOCKED WARD WHERE THE PATIENTS CANNOT COME AND GO AS THEY PLEASE.

5

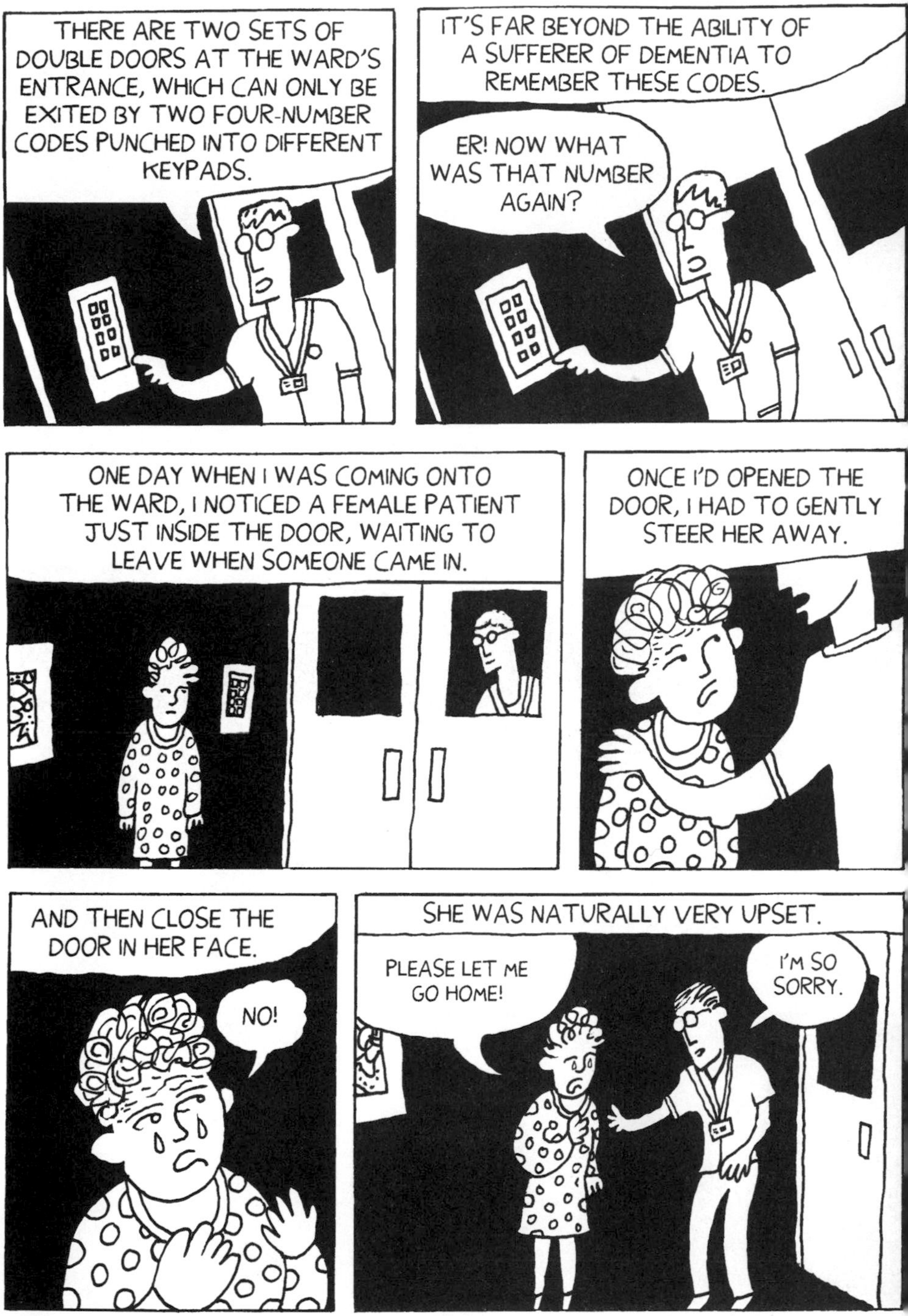
THERE ARE TWO SETS OF DOUBLE DOORS AT THE WARD'S ENTRANCE, WHICH CAN ONLY BE EXITED BY TWO FOUR-NUMBER CODES PUNCHED INTO DIFFERENT KEYPADS.
IT'S FAR BEYOND THE ABILITY OF A SUFFERER OF DEMENTIA TO REMEMBER THESE CODES.
ER! NOW WHAT WAS THAT NUMBER AGAIN?
ONE DAY WHEN I WAS COMING ONTO THE WARD, I NOTICED A FEMALE PATIENT JUST INSIDE THE DOOR, WAITING TO LEAVE WHEN SOMEONE CAME IN.
ONCE I'D OPENED THE DOOR, I HAD TO GENTLY STEER HER AWAY.
AND THEN CLOSE THE DOOR IN HER FACE.
NO!
SHE WAS NATURALLY VERY UPSET.
PLEASE LET ME GO HOME!
I'M SO SORRY.

THERE WAS A PARTICULAR TRAGEDY ABOUT THIS PATIENT, AS SHE WAS STILL QUITE YOUNG.

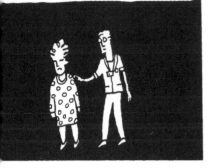

ONLY SIXTY, SHE HAD BEEN DIAGNOSED WITH ALZHEIMER'S DISEASE WHEN SHE WAS FIFTY-FIVE.

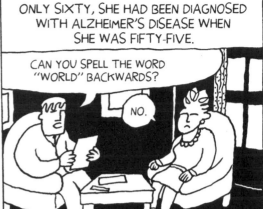

CAN YOU SPELL THE WORD "WORLD" BACKWARDS?

NO.

A MARRIED LADY WHOSE HUSBAND HAD BECOME UNABLE TO CARE FOR HER ANY LONGER.

SOB!

LIKE MANY SHE WAS LIVING ON THE WARD UNTIL A PLACE BECAME AVAILABLE IN A CARE HOME.

BROUGHT YOUR TABLETS.

SHE COULD BECOME VERY AGITATED AT TIMES, BERATING HERSELF WHEN SHE COULDN'T COMPLETE A TASK.

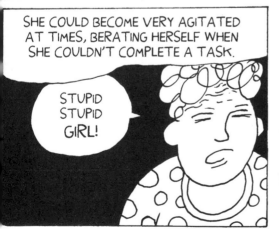

STUPID STUPID GIRL!

HER MEMORY WAS POOR AND SHE NEEDED CONSTANT PROMPTING.

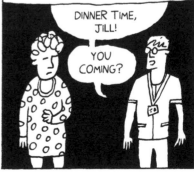

DINNER TIME, JILL!

YOU COMING?

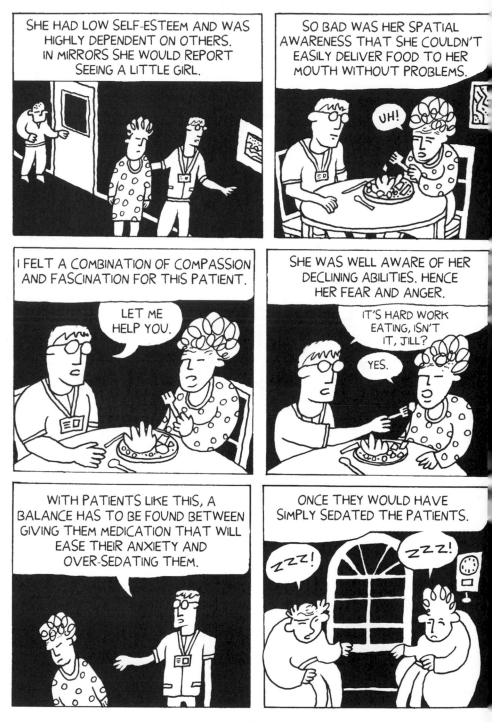

8

BUT NOW QUALITY OF LIFE IS SEEN AS MORE IMPORTANT, EVEN IF THIS MAKES IT DIFFICULT FOR THE STAFF.

HEY!

INCONTINENCE IS, OF COURSE, A BIG ISSUE ON THE DEMENTIA WARD.

WE BETTER TAKE JIM TO THE TOILET.

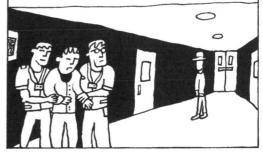

IT'S NOT NICE TO HAVE TO WIPE SOMEONE ELSE'S BOTTOM, BUT SOMEBODY HAS TO DO IT.

ONE DAY, I WAS HELPING A STAFF NURSE ASSIST A PATIENT TO THE TOILET WHEN WE SPIED ANOTHER PATIENT TAKING HIS TROUSERS DOWN IN THE CORRIDOR.

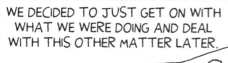

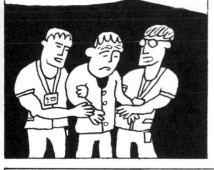

WE DECIDED TO JUST GET ON WITH WHAT WE WERE DOING AND DEAL WITH THIS OTHER MATTER LATER.

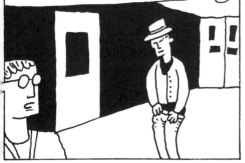

TOILETING CAN BE A PROBLEM ON THE DEMENTIA WARD.

NO!

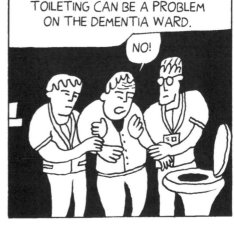

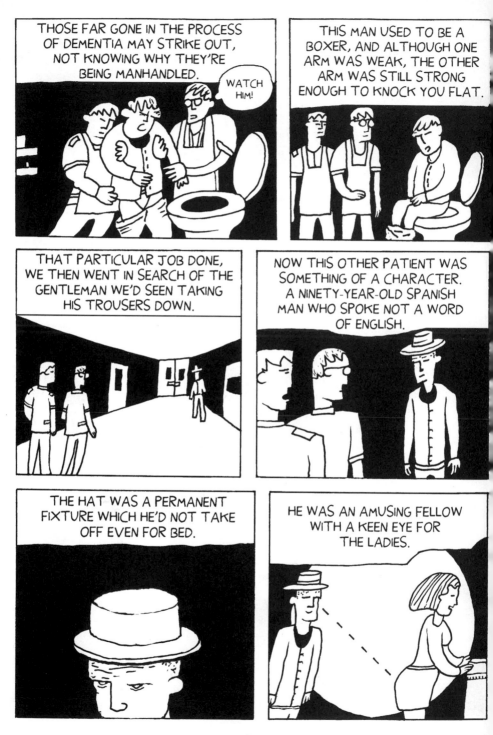

10

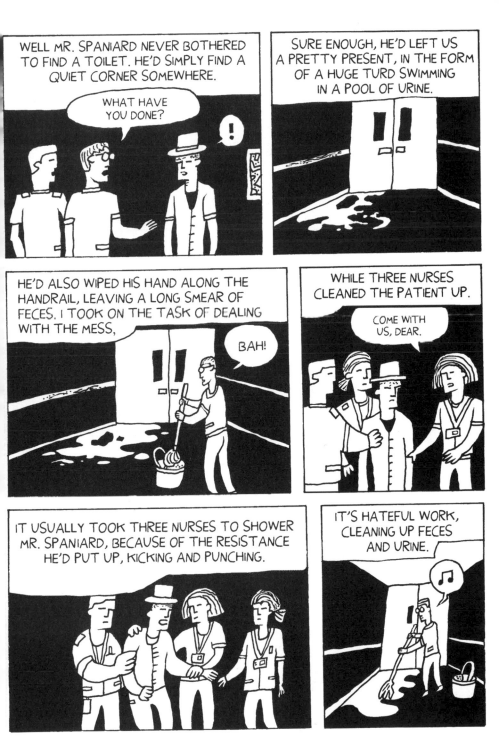

11

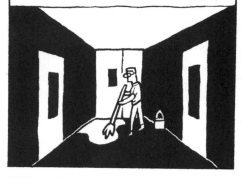

HOWEVER, IT'S BASIC NURSING AND IF YOU CAN'T DO IT, THEN YOU SHOULDN'T BE A NURSE.

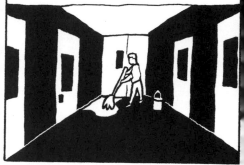

DEMENTIA PATIENTS ARE LIKE CHILDREN. YOU HAVE TO WATCH THEM ALL THE TIME.

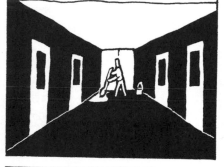

ON ONE OCCASION THE SPANISH PATIENT HAD LEFT A BOWEL MOVEMENT IN THE CORRIDOR.

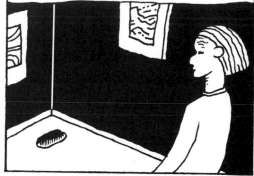

BY THE TIME THE TURD WAS DISCOVERED,

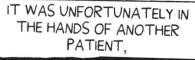

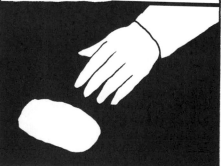

IT WAS UNFORTUNATELY IN THE HANDS OF ANOTHER PATIENT,

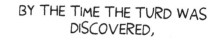

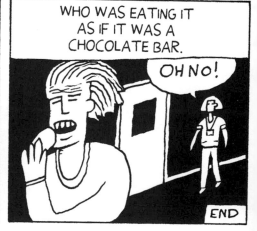

WHO WAS EATING IT AS IF IT WAS A CHOCOLATE BAR.

OH NO!

END

12

cut

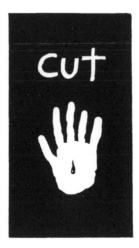

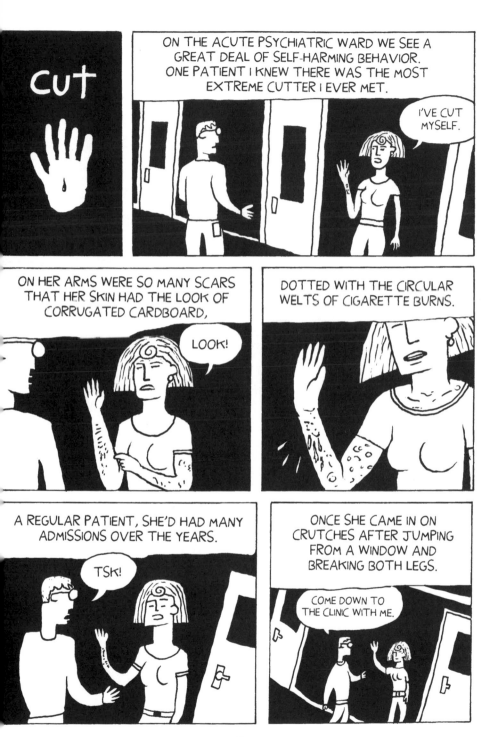

CUT

ON THE ACUTE PSYCHIATRIC WARD WE SEE A GREAT DEAL OF SELF-HARMING BEHAVIOR. ONE PATIENT I KNEW THERE WAS THE MOST EXTREME CUTTER I EVER MET.

I'VE CUT MYSELF.

ON HER ARMS WERE SO MANY SCARS THAT HER SKIN HAD THE LOOK OF CORRUGATED CARDBOARD,

LOOK!

DOTTED WITH THE CIRCULAR WELTS OF CIGARETTE BURNS.

A REGULAR PATIENT, SHE'D HAD MANY ADMISSIONS OVER THE YEARS.

TSK!

ONCE SHE CAME IN ON CRUTCHES AFTER JUMPING FROM A WINDOW AND BREAKING BOTH LEGS.

COME DOWN TO THE CLINIC WITH ME.

17

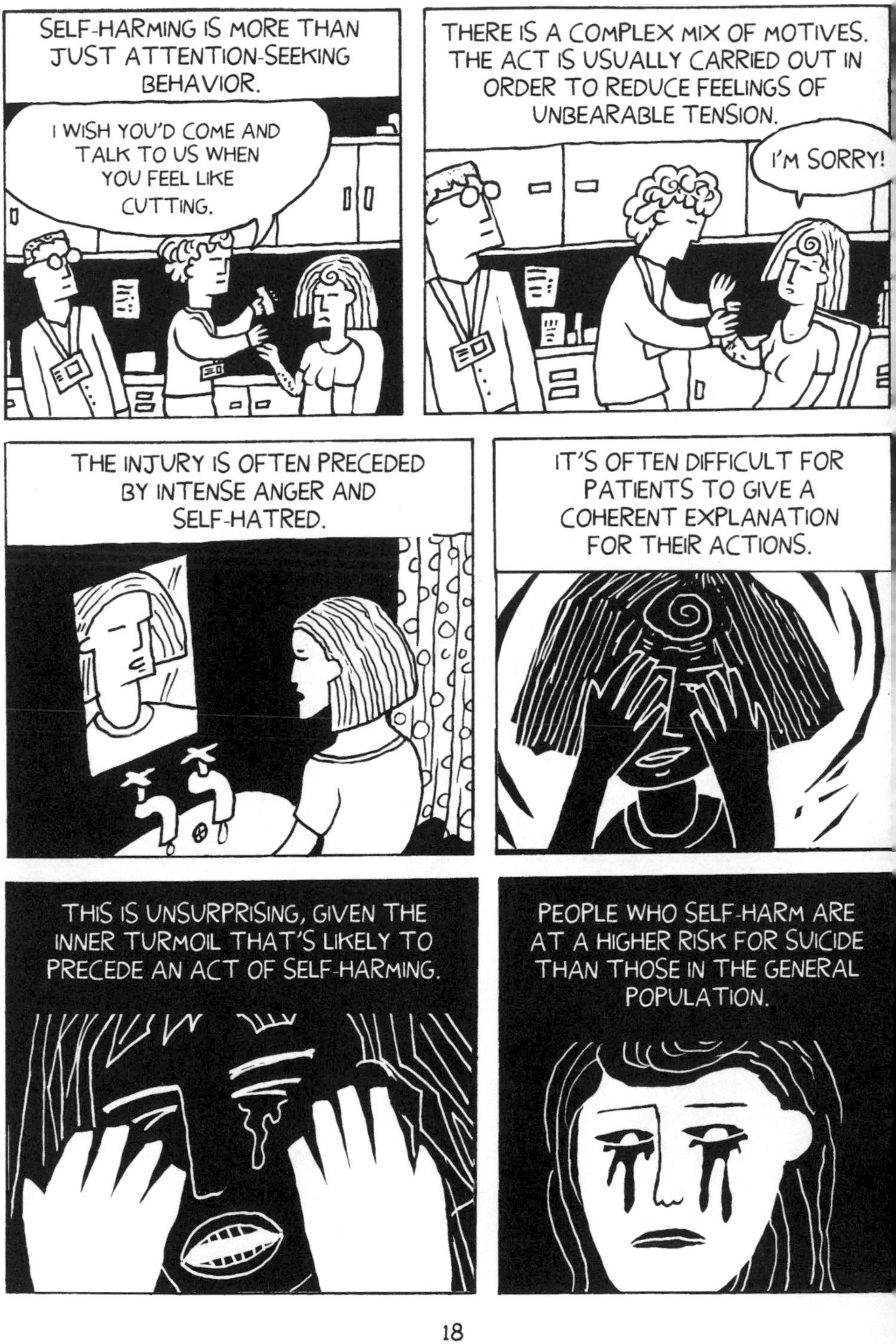
SELF-HARMING IS MORE THAN JUST ATTENTION-SEEKING BEHAVIOR.
I WISH YOU'D COME AND TALK TO US WHEN YOU FEEL LIKE CUTTING.
THERE IS A COMPLEX MIX OF MOTIVES. THE ACT IS USUALLY CARRIED OUT IN ORDER TO REDUCE FEELINGS OF UNBEARABLE TENSION.
I'M SORRY!
THE INJURY IS OFTEN PRECEDED BY INTENSE ANGER AND SELF-HATRED.
IT'S OFTEN DIFFICULT FOR PATIENTS TO GIVE A COHERENT EXPLANATION FOR THEIR ACTIONS.
THIS IS UNSURPRISING, GIVEN THE INNER TURMOIL THAT'S LIKELY TO PRECEDE AN ACT OF SELF-HARMING.
PEOPLE WHO SELF-HARM ARE AT A HIGHER RISK FOR SUICIDE THAN THOSE IN THE GENERAL POPULATION.

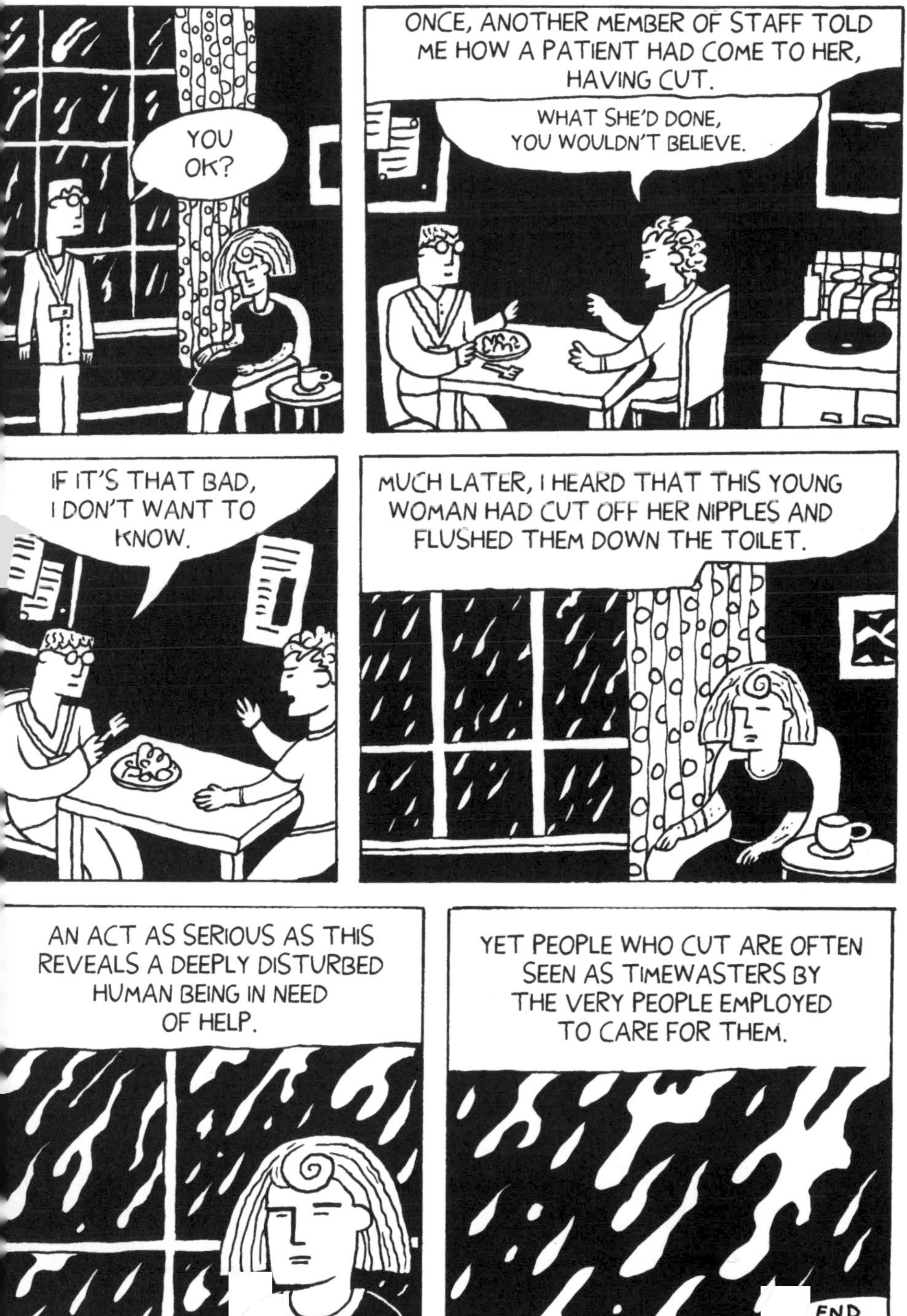
YOU OK?
ONCE, ANOTHER MEMBER OF STAFF TOLD ME HOW A PATIENT HAD COME TO HER, HAVING CUT.
WHAT SHE'D DONE, YOU WOULDN'T BELIEVE.
IF IT'S THAT BAD, I DON'T WANT TO KNOW.
MUCH LATER, I HEARD THAT THIS YOUNG WOMAN HAD CUT OFF HER NIPPLES AND FLUSHED THEM DOWN THE TOILET.
AN ACT AS SERIOUS AS THIS REVEALS A DEEPLY DISTURBED HUMAN BEING IN NEED OF HELP.
YET PEOPLE WHO CUT ARE OFTEN SEEN AS TIMEWASTERS BY THE VERY PEOPLE EMPLOYED TO CARE FOR THEM.
END

IT
COULD
BE
YOU

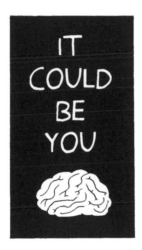

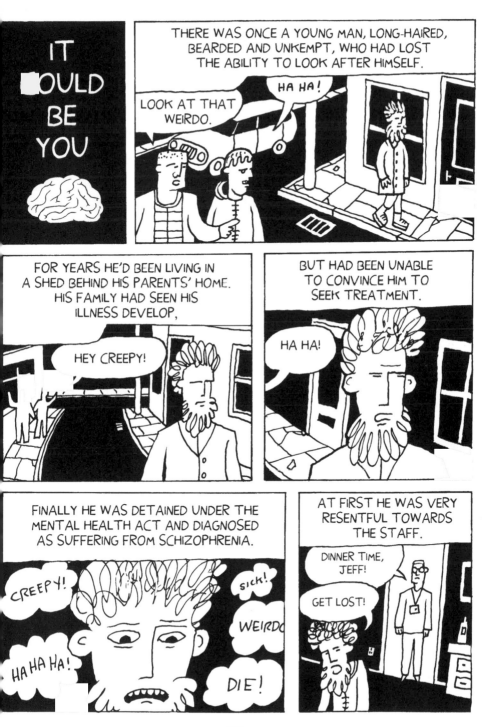

23

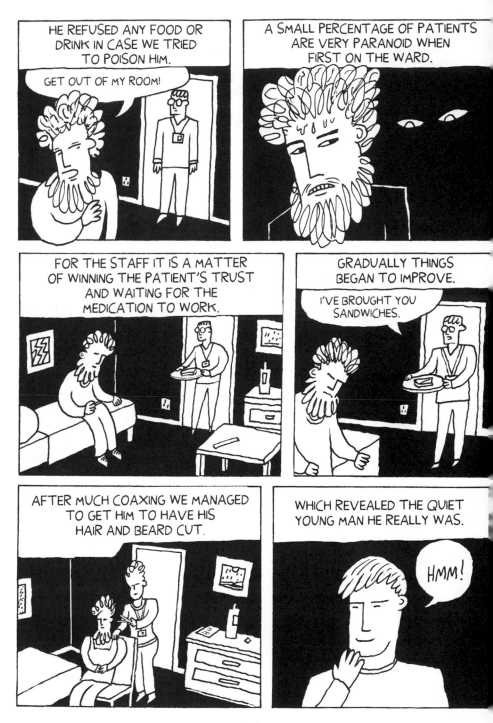

24

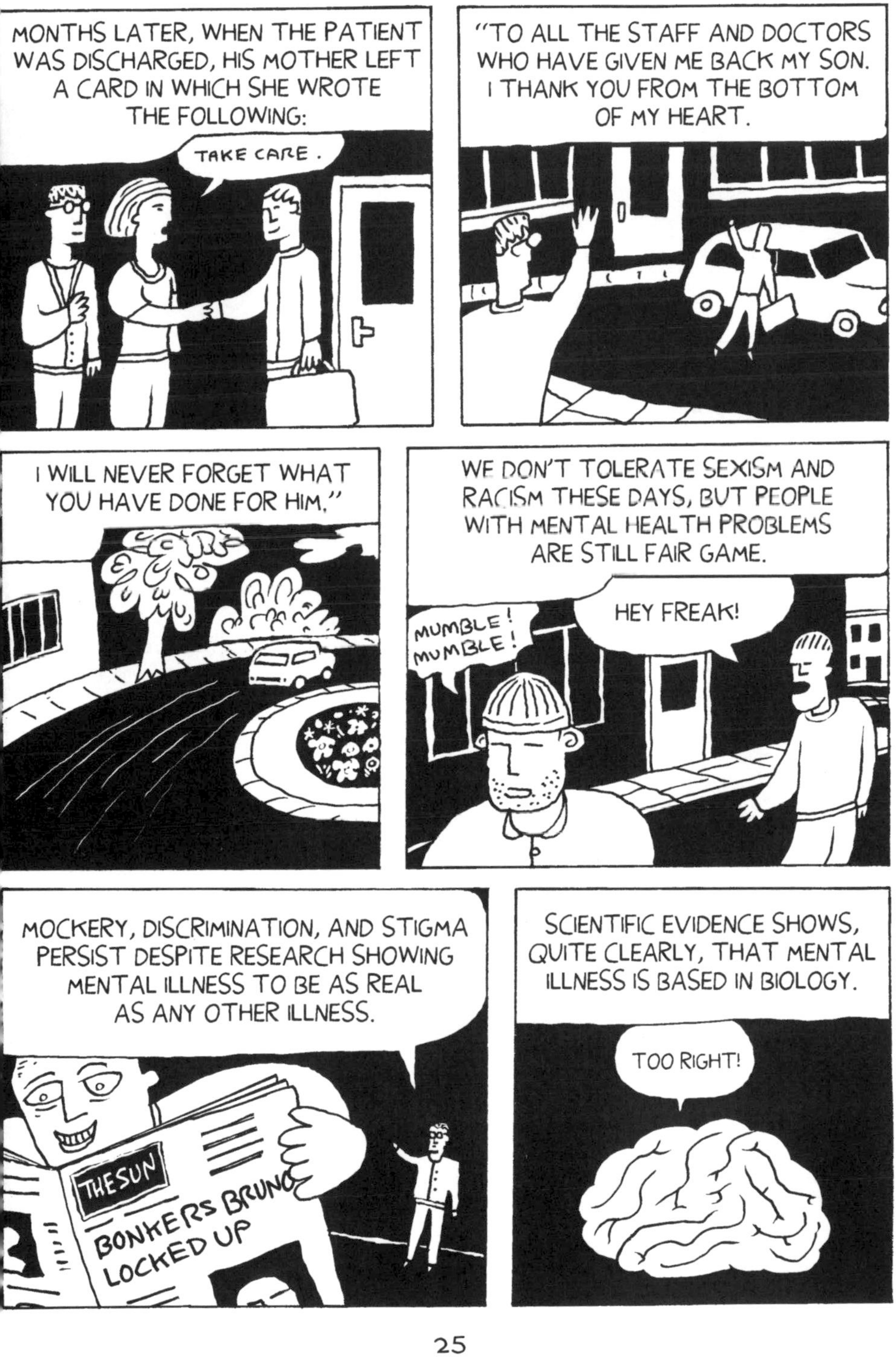

MONTHS LATER, WHEN THE PATIENT WAS DISCHARGED, HIS MOTHER LEFT A CARD IN WHICH SHE WROTE THE FOLLOWING:

TAKE CARE.

"TO ALL THE STAFF AND DOCTORS WHO HAVE GIVEN ME BACK MY SON. I THANK YOU FROM THE BOTTOM OF MY HEART.

I WILL NEVER FORGET WHAT YOU HAVE DONE FOR HIM."

WE DON'T TOLERATE SEXISM AND RACISM THESE DAYS, BUT PEOPLE WITH MENTAL HEALTH PROBLEMS ARE STILL FAIR GAME.

MUMBLE! MUMBLE!

HEY FREAK!

MOCKERY, DISCRIMINATION, AND STIGMA PERSIST DESPITE RESEARCH SHOWING MENTAL ILLNESS TO BE AS REAL AS ANY OTHER ILLNESS.

THE SUN

BONKERS BRUNO LOCKED UP

SCIENTIFIC EVIDENCE SHOWS, QUITE CLEARLY, THAT MENTAL ILLNESS IS BASED IN BIOLOGY.

TOO RIGHT!

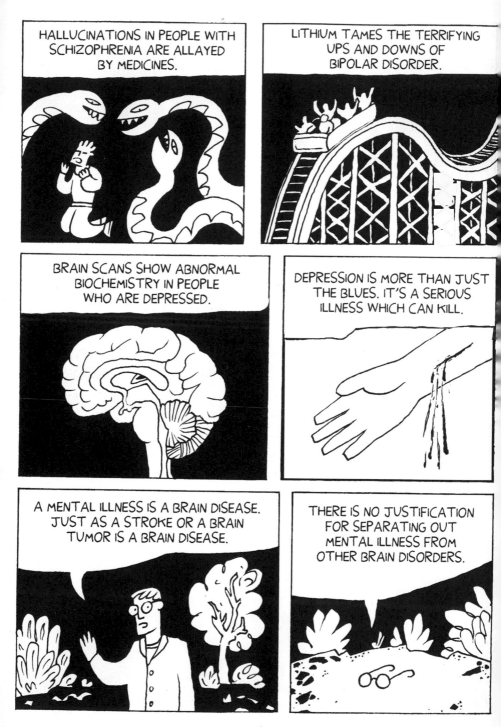

HALLUCINATIONS IN PEOPLE WITH SCHIZOPHRENIA ARE ALLAYED BY MEDICINES.

LITHIUM TAMES THE TERRIFYING UPS AND DOWNS OF BIPOLAR DISORDER.

BRAIN SCANS SHOW ABNORMAL BIOCHEMISTRY IN PEOPLE WHO ARE DEPRESSED.

DEPRESSION IS MORE THAN JUST THE BLUES. IT'S A SERIOUS ILLNESS WHICH CAN KILL.

A MENTAL ILLNESS IS A BRAIN DISEASE. JUST AS A STROKE OR A BRAIN TUMOR IS A BRAIN DISEASE.

THERE IS NO JUSTIFICATION FOR SEPARATING OUT MENTAL ILLNESS FROM OTHER BRAIN DISORDERS.

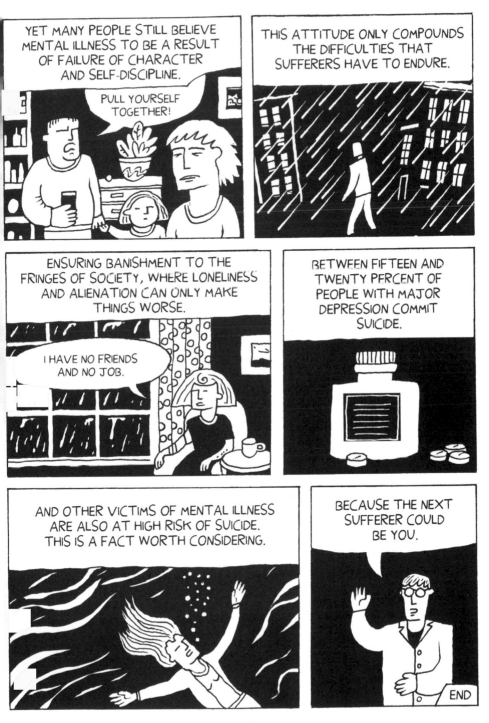

27

DARKNESS

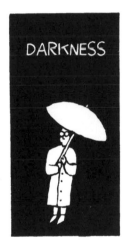

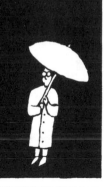

DARKNESS

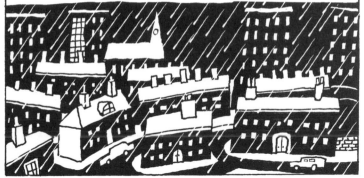

NO ONE HAS TO BE TAUGHT HOW TO BE DEPRESSED AS EVERYONE HAS EXPERIENCED SOME LEVEL OF DEPRESSION IN THEIR LIVES.

HOWEVER, THERE IS A DIFFERENCE BETWEEN EVERYDAY SADNESS AND THE CHRONIC DEPRESSION WHICH CAN AFFECT SUFFERERS FOR YEARS.

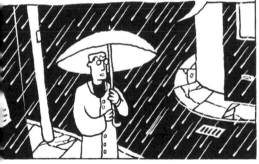

I REMEMBER A FEMALE PATIENT BEING ADMITTED TO THE WARD. HER HUSBAND SAT IN DURING THE FORM-FILLING.

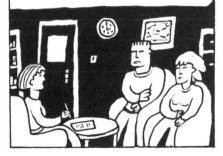

A SWAGGERING BULLY, THIS MAN BELITTLED HIS WIFE EVEN AS SHE WAS BEING ADMITTED INTO THE HOSPITAL.

SHE DOES NOTHING AROUND THE HOUSE.

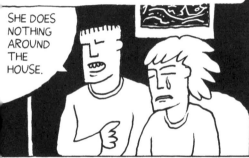

I FEEL SO WORTHLESS. I CAN'T SLEEP AND I'M INTERESTED IN NOTHING.

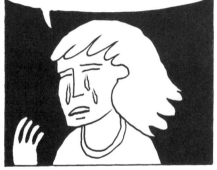

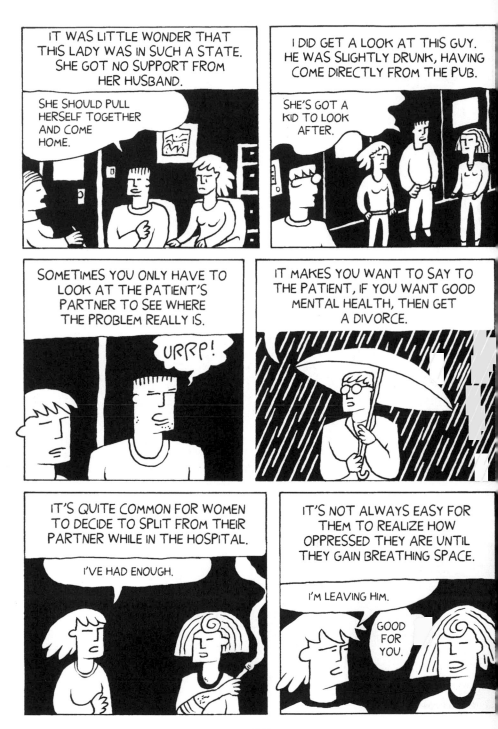

32

DEPRESSION ISN'T JUST A BLUE MOOD YOU CAN JUST SNAP OUT OF. IT'S A SERIOUS BIOLOGICAL ILLNESS,

FOR YEARS I'VE HAD NO LIFE OF MY OWN.

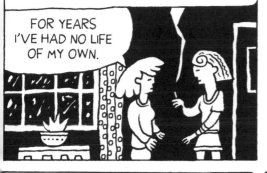

WHICH AFFECTS BEHAVIOR, THOUGHTS, AND FEELINGS.

I KNOW EXACTLY WHAT YOU MEAN, DEAR.

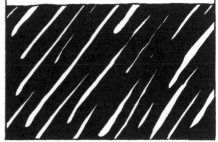

IN THE BRAIN THERE ARE NATURALLY OCCURRING SUBSTANCES CALLED NEUROTRANSMITTERS.

WILL THIS RAIN EVER STOP?

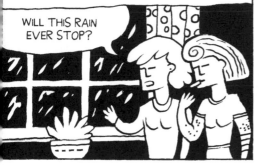

THESE ARE THE CHEMICAL MESSENGERS THAT CARRY ELECTRICAL SIGNALS FROM ONE NERVE CELL TO ANOTHER,

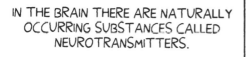

ACROSS SPACES CALLED SYNAPSES.

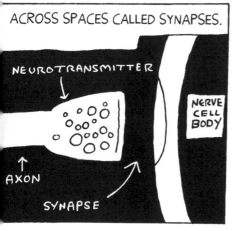

NEUROTRANSMITTER

NERVE CELL BODY

AXON

SYNAPSE

THE NEUROTRANSMITTERS THAT PLAY A SIGNIFICANT ROLE IN MAINTAINING OUR MOOD ARE SEROTONIN AND NOREPINEPHRINE.

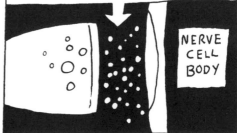

NERVE CELL BODY

IT'S WHEN THESE NEUROTRANSMITTERS ARE AT LOW LEVELS THAT THE VEGETATIVE SYMPTOMS OF DEPRESSION BECOME CLINICALLY EVIDENT.

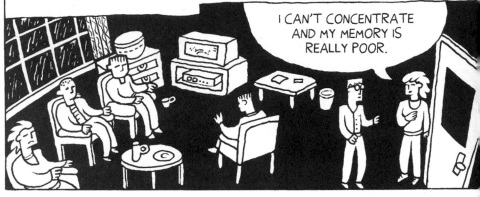

I CAN'T CONCENTRATE AND MY MEMORY IS REALLY POOR.

DEPRESSION MAKES THINKING SLUGGISH. ANTIDEPRESSANTS HELP TO RESTORE THE BALANCE OF NEUROTRANSMITTERS IN THE BRAIN,

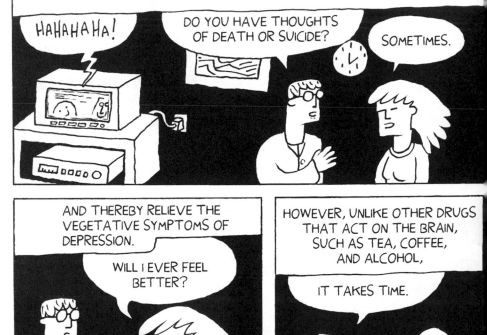

HAHAHAHA!

DO YOU HAVE THOUGHTS OF DEATH OR SUICIDE?

SOMETIMES.

AND THEREBY RELIEVE THE VEGETATIVE SYMPTOMS OF DEPRESSION.

WILL I EVER FEEL BETTER?

HOWEVER, UNLIKE OTHER DRUGS THAT ACT ON THE BRAIN, SUCH AS TEA, COFFEE, AND ALCOHOL,

IT TAKES TIME.

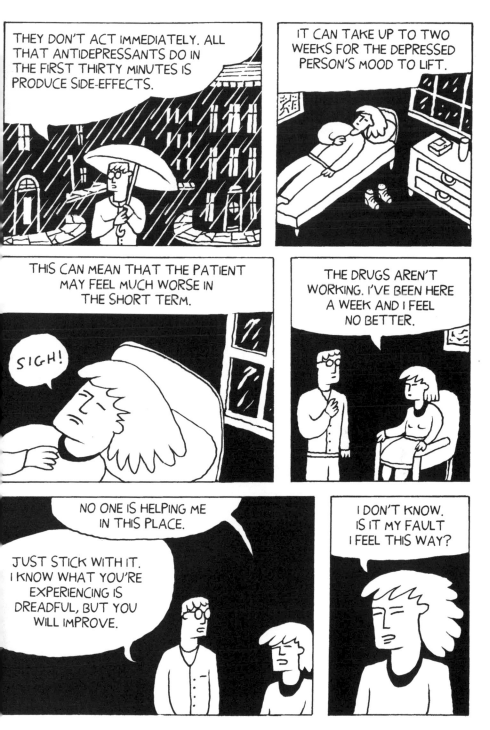

35

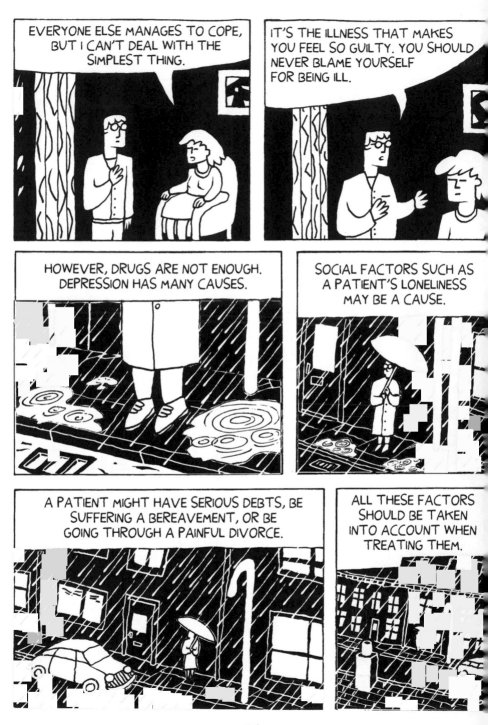

THERE ARE ADVOCACY SERVICES FOR THOSE WHO NEED HELP WITH SUCH PROBLEMS AS DEBT OR HOUSING. THERE ARE SOCIAL VENUES WHICH HAVE BEEN SET UP TO CATER TO THOSE WHO SUFFER FROM PSYCHIATRIC ILLNESSES.

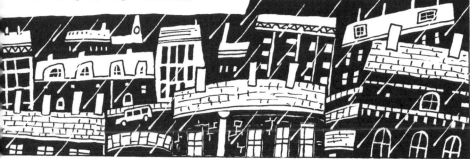

AS WELL AS PSYCHOTHERAPY FOR THOSE WHO NEED TO RESOLVE LIFE PROBLEMS.

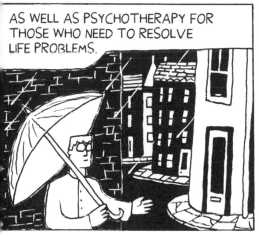

THE FEELINGS OF DESPAIR AND HELPLESSNESS THAT DEPRESSION BRINGS

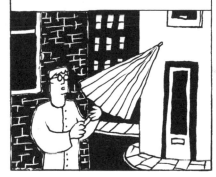

CAN BE ALLEVIATED THROUGH PROPER CARE AND TREATMENT. IT'S MORE THAN POSSIBLE TO LIVE A FULFILLING LIFE DESPITE THE ILLNESS.

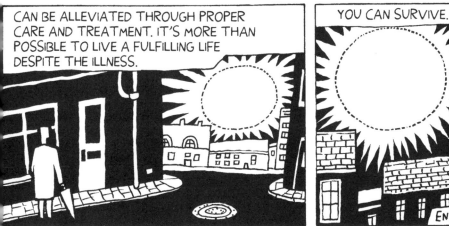

YOU CAN SURVIVE.

END

ANTI-SOCIAL PERSONALITY DISORDER
GRR!

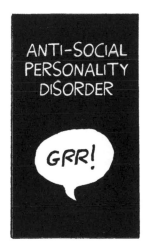

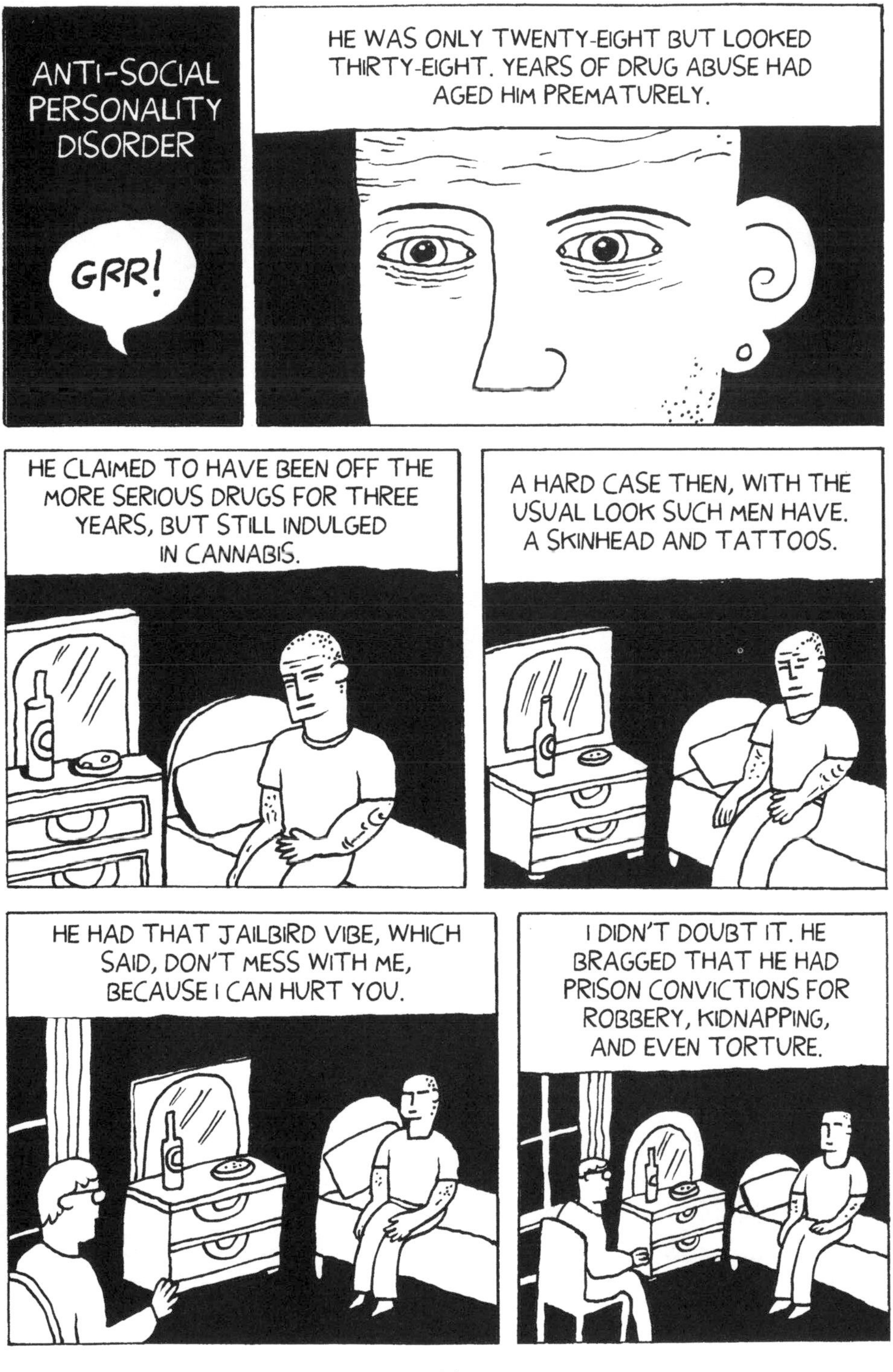

ANTI-SOCIAL PERSONALITY DISORDER
GRR!
HE WAS ONLY TWENTY-EIGHT BUT LOOKED THIRTY-EIGHT. YEARS OF DRUG ABUSE HAD AGED HIM PREMATURELY.
HE CLAIMED TO HAVE BEEN OFF THE MORE SERIOUS DRUGS FOR THREE YEARS, BUT STILL INDULGED IN CANNABIS.
A HARD CASE THEN, WITH THE USUAL LOOK SUCH MEN HAVE. A SKINHEAD AND TATTOOS.
HE HAD THAT JAILBIRD VIBE, WHICH SAID, DON'T MESS WITH ME, BECAUSE I CAN HURT YOU.
I DIDN'T DOUBT IT. HE BRAGGED THAT HE HAD PRISON CONVICTIONS FOR ROBBERY, KIDNAPPING, AND EVEN TORTURE.

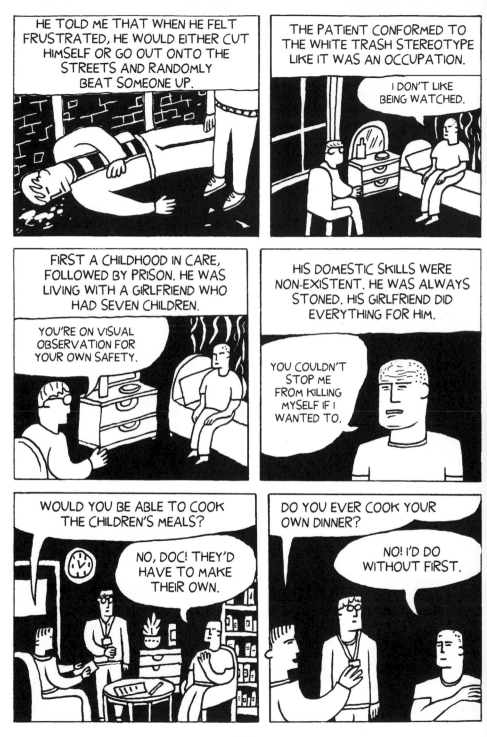

42

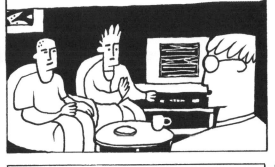

HE'D BEEN ARRESTED ON A MUGGING CHARGE AND THEN SENT TO US FOR PSYCHIATRIC EVALUATION. HE CLAIMED TO BE SUICIDAL.

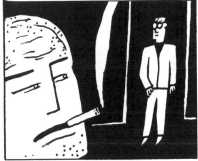

THIS IS A FAMILIAR PATTERN WITH THOSE PATIENTS IN TROUBLE WITH THE LAW.

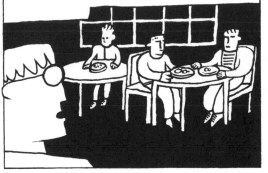

THEY THINK THEY'LL RECEIVE A LESSER SENTENCE IF THEY CAN CONVINCE THE COURTS THAT THEY SUFFER A MENTAL ILLNESS. IT RARELY WORKS.

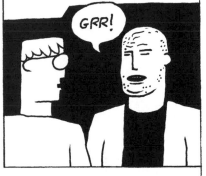

HE WAS A FRIGHTENING CHARACTER WHO SCARED ME MORE THAN ANY PATIENT I EVER MET.

GRR!

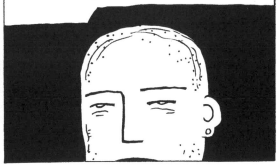

THIS WAS IN THE TIME BEFORE WE BEGAN TO USE PERSONAL ALARMS. I WAS NERVOUS AS HELL, SHADOWING A MAN WHO WAS SO HOSTILE.

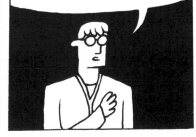

THE NEXT DAY, AS WE'D SEEN NO EVIDENCE OF DEPRESSION, HE WAS REGRADED TO THIRTY MINUTES OBSERVATION.

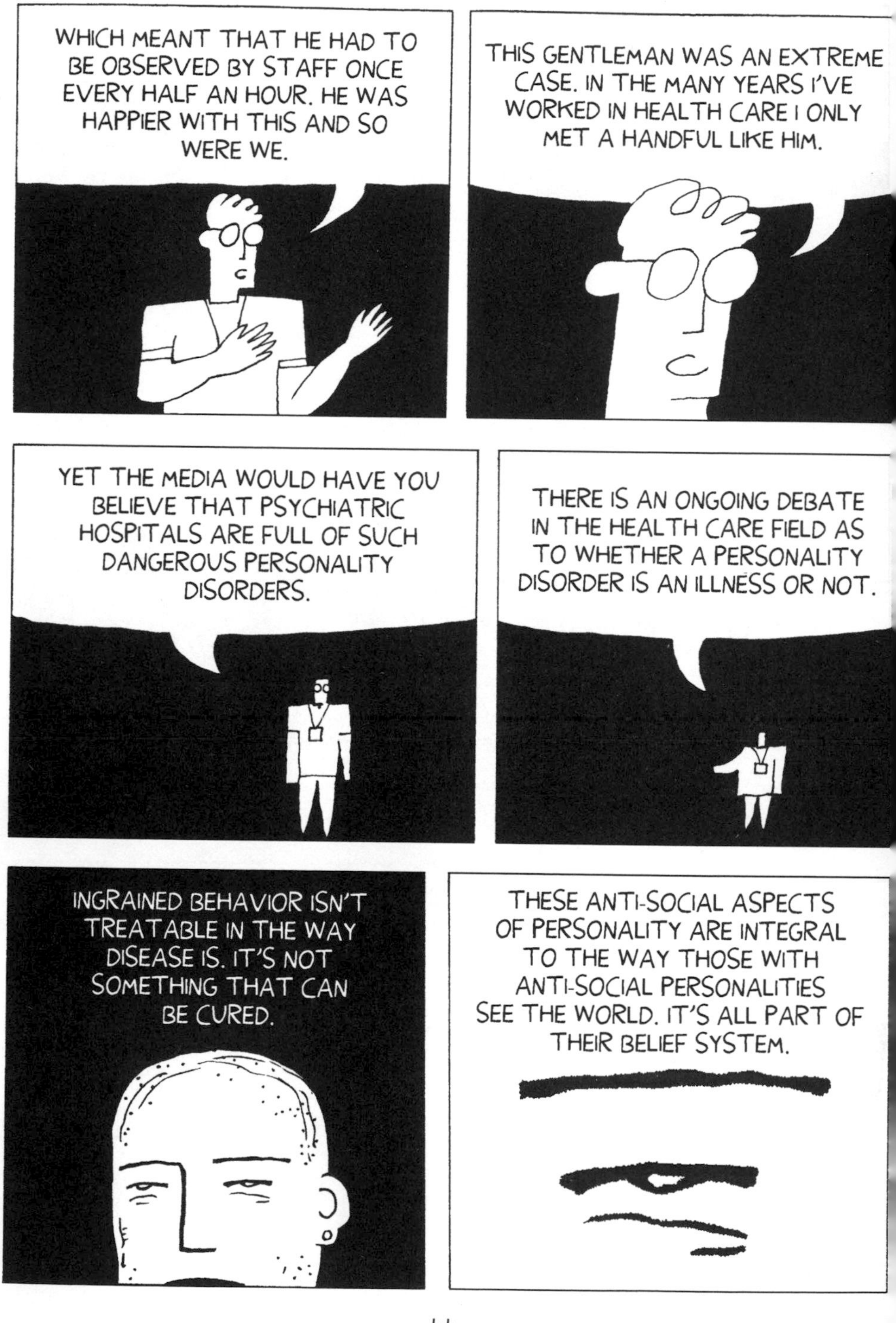

WHICH MEANT THAT HE HAD TO BE OBSERVED BY STAFF ONCE EVERY HALF AN HOUR. HE WAS HAPPIER WITH THIS AND SO WERE WE.

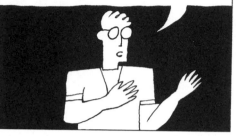

THIS GENTLEMAN WAS AN EXTREME CASE. IN THE MANY YEARS I'VE WORKED IN HEALTH CARE I ONLY MET A HANDFUL LIKE HIM.

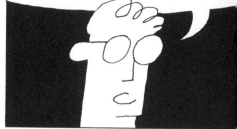

YET THE MEDIA WOULD HAVE YOU BELIEVE THAT PSYCHIATRIC HOSPITALS ARE FULL OF SUCH DANGEROUS PERSONALITY DISORDERS.

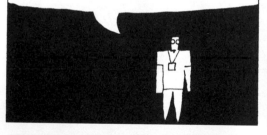

THERE IS AN ONGOING DEBATE IN THE HEALTH CARE FIELD AS TO WHETHER A PERSONALITY DISORDER IS AN ILLNESS OR NOT.

INGRAINED BEHAVIOR ISN'T TREATABLE IN THE WAY DISEASE IS. IT'S NOT SOMETHING THAT CAN BE CURED.

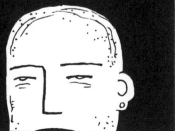

THESE ANTI-SOCIAL ASPECTS OF PERSONALITY ARE INTEGRAL TO THE WAY THOSE WITH ANTI-SOCIAL PERSONALITIES SEE THE WORLD. IT'S ALL PART OF THEIR BELIEF SYSTEM.

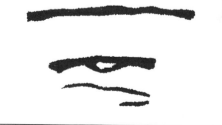

44

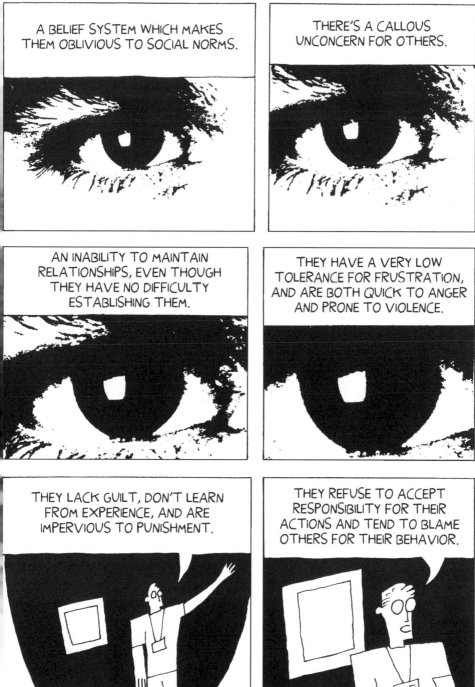

45

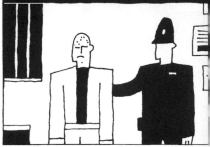

I DON'T KNOW WHAT HAPPENED TO THIS PATIENT. I WENT ON HOLIDAY AND WHEN I RETURNED HE WAS GONE.

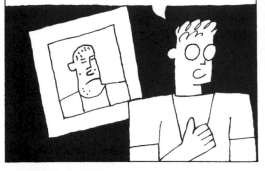

I PRESUMED THAT HAVING BEEN ASSESSED HE'D BEEN TAKEN BACK INTO CUSTODY.

NOT ALL PEOPLE WITH THIS TYPE OF PERSONALITY DISORDER ARE CRIMINALS.

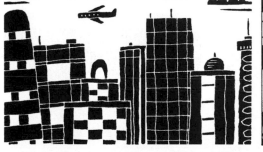

WE LIVE IN A SOCIETY WHERE MANY OF THESE PSYCHOPATHIC TRAITS ARE CONSIDERED QUITE REASONABLE.

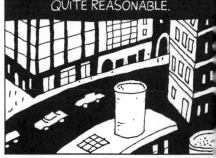

SELFISHNESS, LACK OF EMPATHY, SUPERFICIALITY, AND MANIPULATIVENESS

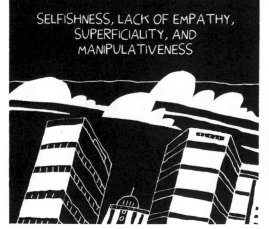

ARE TRAITS THAT ARE HIGHLY VALUED IN THE WORLDS OF BUSINESS, POLITICS, THE LAW, AND ACADEMIA.

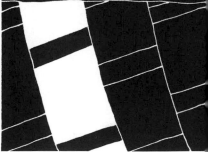

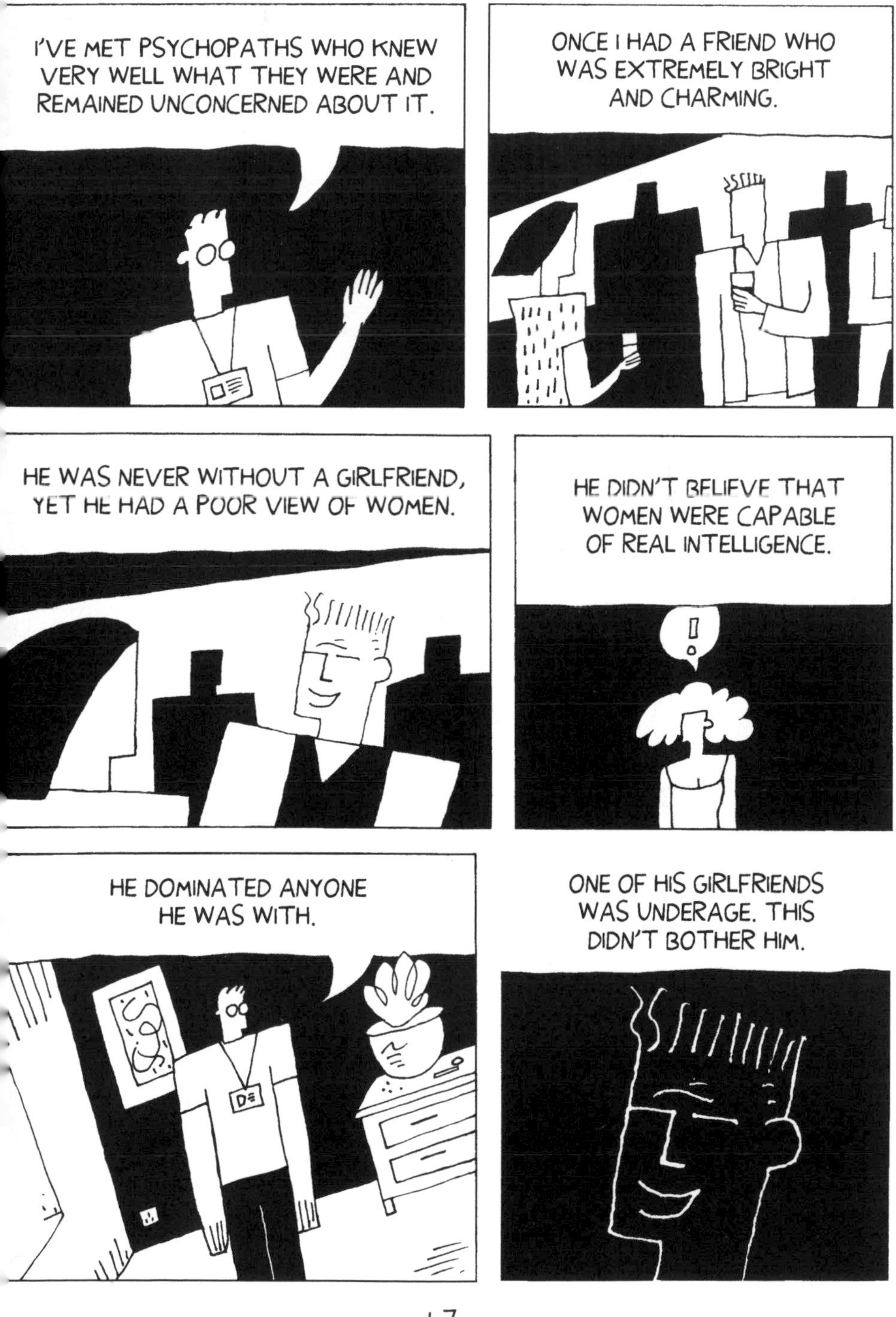

I'VE MET PSYCHOPATHS WHO KNEW VERY WELL WHAT THEY WERE AND REMAINED UNCONCERNED ABOUT IT.

ONCE I HAD A FRIEND WHO WAS EXTREMELY BRIGHT AND CHARMING.

HE WAS NEVER WITHOUT A GIRLFRIEND, YET HE HAD A POOR VIEW OF WOMEN.

HE DIDN'T BELIEVE THAT WOMEN WERE CAPABLE OF REAL INTELLIGENCE.

HE DOMINATED ANYONE HE WAS WITH.

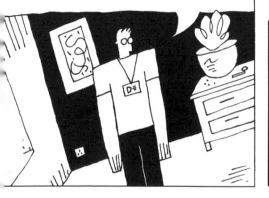

ONE OF HIS GIRLFRIENDS WAS UNDERAGE. THIS DIDN'T BOTHER HIM.

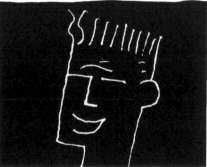

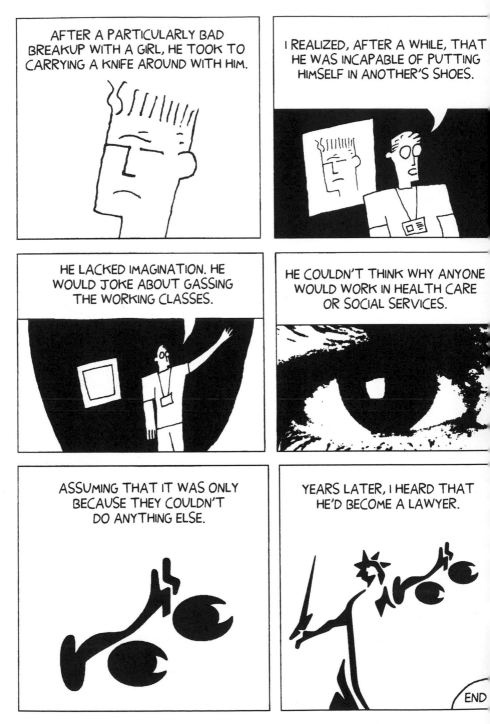

48

PEOPLE
WITH
MENTAL
ILLNESS
ENRICH
OUR
LIVES

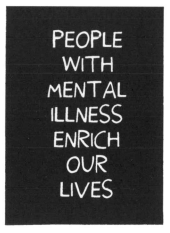

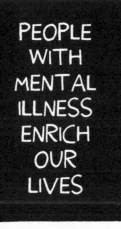

PEOPLE WITH MENTAL ILLNESS ENRICH OUR LIVES

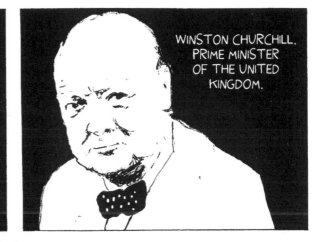

WINSTON CHURCHILL. PRIME MINISTER OF THE UNITED KINGDOM.

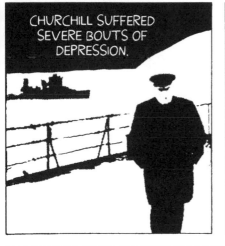

CHURCHILL SUFFERED SEVERE BOUTS OF DEPRESSION.

WHICH HE REFERRED TO AS HIS BLACK DOG.

HE HAD MANY OF THE TRAITS WE NOW ASSOCIATE WITH BIPOLAR DISORDER.

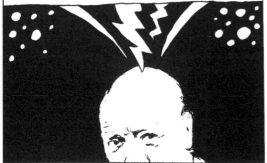

BELLIGERENCE, ABNORMAL ENERGY, LACK OF INHIBITION, AND GRANDIOSITY.

HAH!

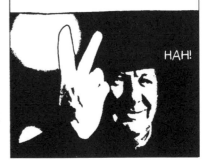

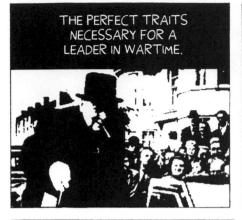

THE PERFECT TRAITS NECESSARY FOR A LEADER IN WARTIME.

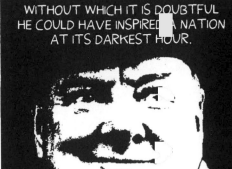

WITHOUT WHICH IT IS DOUBTFUL HE COULD HAVE INSPIRED A NATION AT ITS DARKEST HOUR.

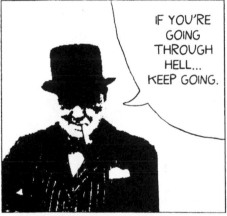

IF YOU'RE GOING THROUGH HELL... KEEP GOING.

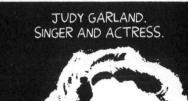

JUDY GARLAND. SINGER AND ACTRESS.

IF I AM A LEGEND, WHY AM I SO LONELY.

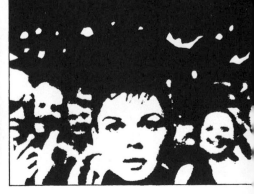

DESPITE SUCCESSFUL FILM AND RECORDING CAREERS, MANY AWARDS, AND HUGE CRITICAL PRAISE

GARLAND SUFFERED THROUGHOUT HER LIFE FROM LACERATING SELF-DOUBT.

SHE REQUIRED CONSTANT REASSURANCE THAT SHE WAS TALENTED AND ATTRACTIVE.

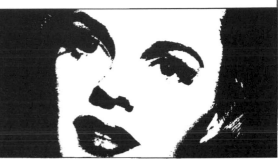

AS A TEENAGE STAR SHE WAS PLIED WITH DRUGS IN ORDER TO KEEP HER WEIGHT DOWN.

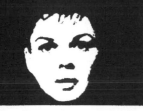

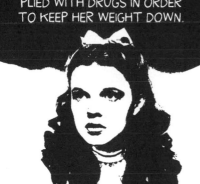

A SITUATION THAT BROUGHT ABOUT A LIFELONG STRUGGLE WITH ADDICTION

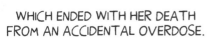

WHICH ENDED WITH HER DEATH FROM AN ACCIDENTAL OVERDOSE.

YET OUT OF THE CHAOS OF HER LIFE, GARLAND LEFT A LASTING LEGACY.

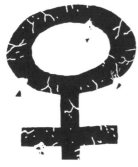

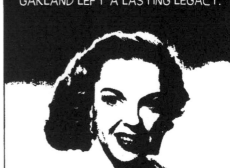

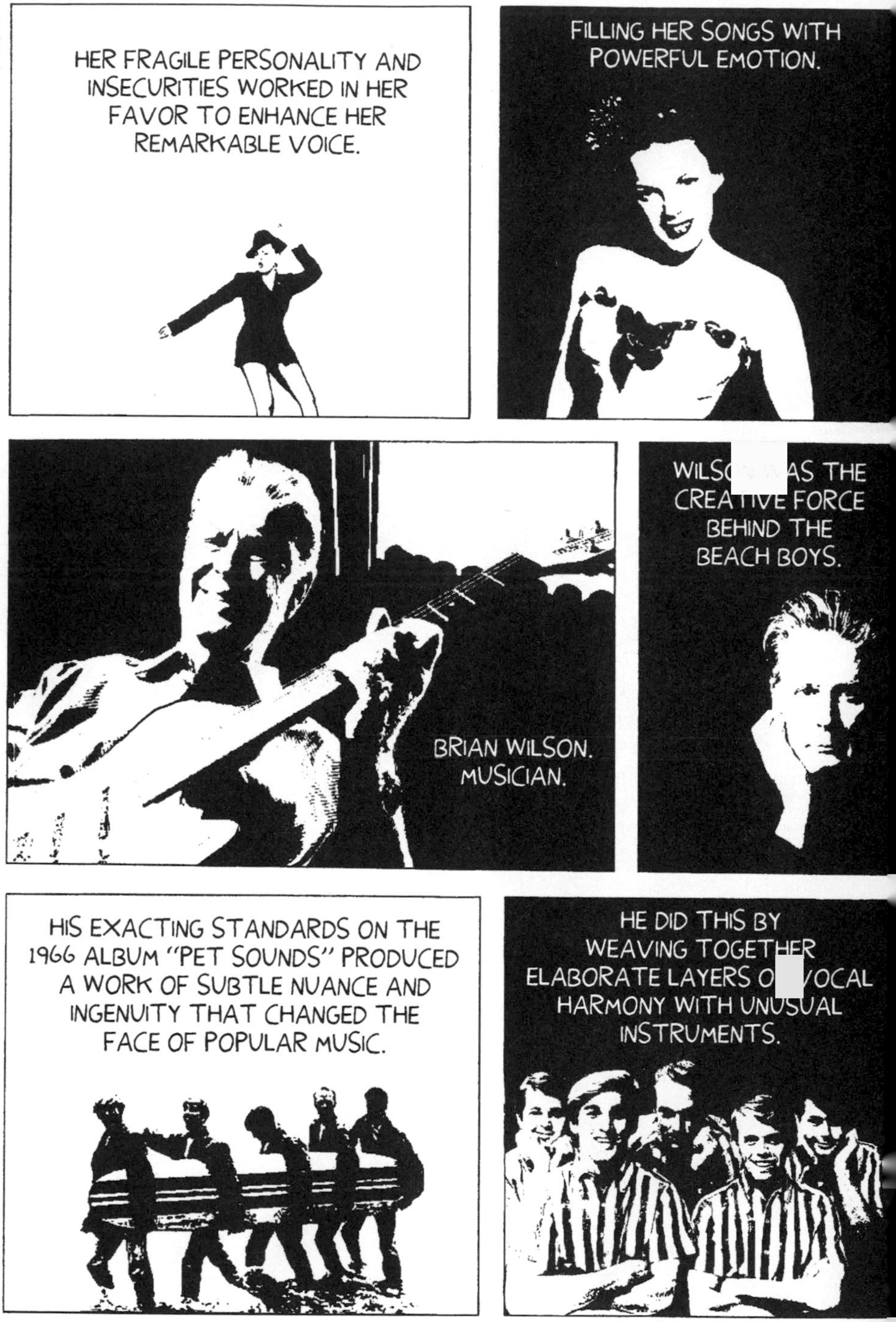
HER FRAGILE PERSONALITY AND INSECURITIES WORKED IN HER FAVOR TO ENHANCE HER REMARKABLE VOICE.
FILLING HER SONGS WITH POWERFUL EMOTION.
BRIAN WILSON. MUSICIAN.
WILSO AS THE CREATIVE FORCE BEHIND THE BEACH BOYS.
HIS EXACTING STANDARDS ON THE 1966 ALBUM "PET SOUNDS" PRODUCED A WORK OF SUBTLE NUANCE AND INGENUITY THAT CHANGED THE FACE OF POPULAR MUSIC.
HE DID THIS BY WEAVING TOGETHER ELABORATE LAYERS O VOCAL HARMONY WITH UNUSUAL INSTRUMENTS.

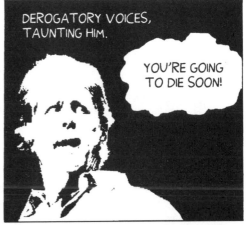

IN HIS MID-TWENTIES, WILSON BEGAN TO EXPERIENCE AUDITORY HALLUCINATIONS.

HEY!

DEROGATORY VOICES, TAUNTING HIM.

YOU'RE GOING TO DIE SOON!

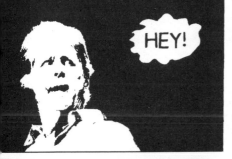

THESE VOICES NEVER LEFT WILSON, MAKING IT IMPOSSIBLE FOR HIM TO GO ON STAGE FOR MANY YEARS.

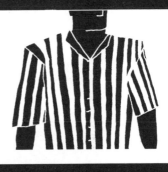

THIS, COMBINED WITH HIS OBSESSIVE PERFECTIONISM, AND THE GROWING TENSIONS WITHIN THE BAND,

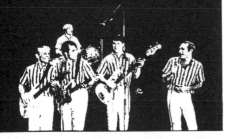

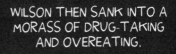

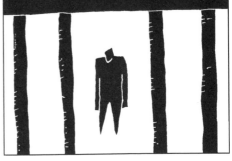

BROUGHT ABOUT AN END TO WILSON'S LEADERSHIP OF THE BEACH BOYS.

WILSON THEN SANK INTO A MORASS OF DRUG-TAKING AND OVEREATING.

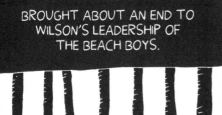

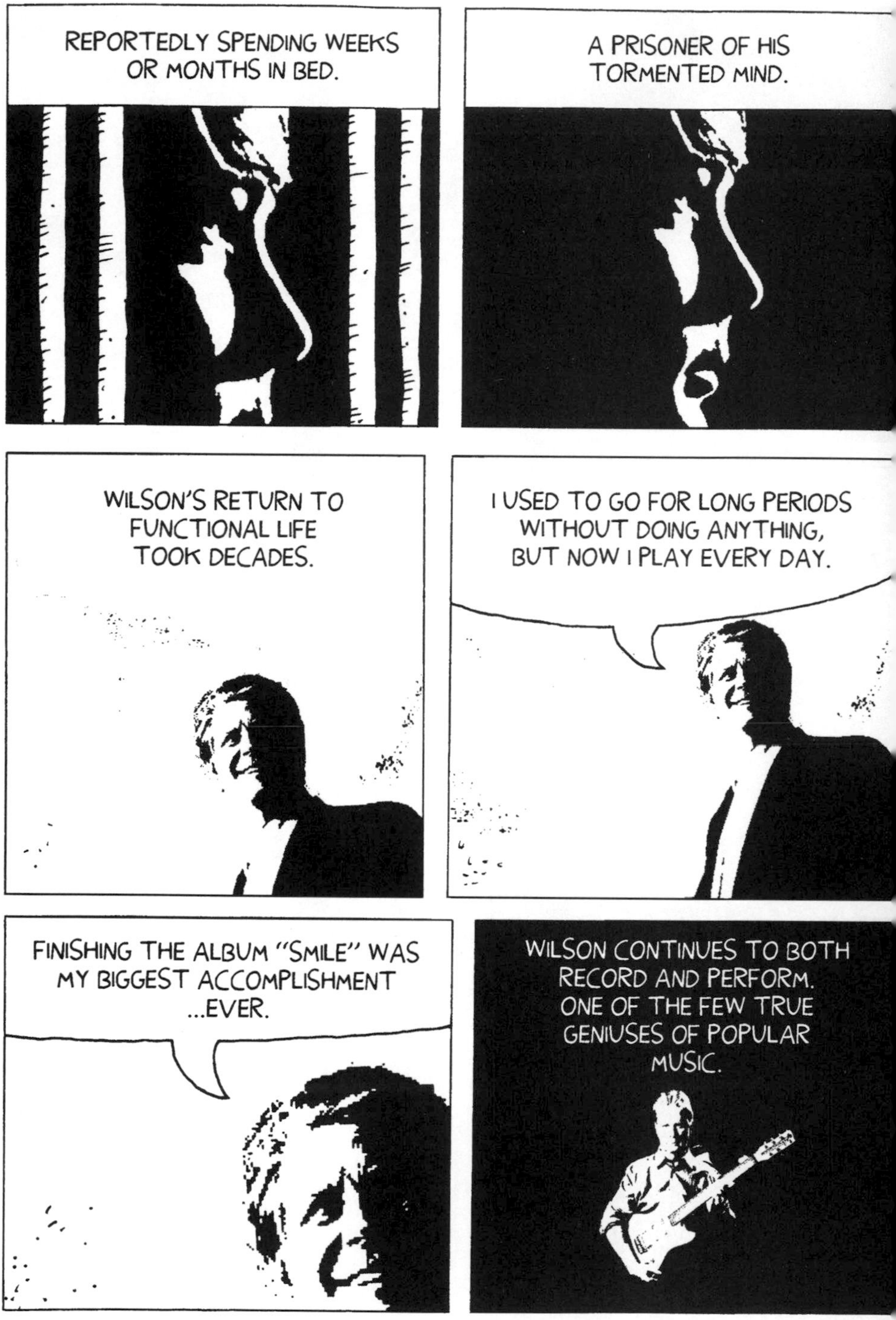
REPORTEDLY SPENDING WEEKS OR MONTHS IN BED.
A PRISONER OF HIS TORMENTED MIND.
WILSON'S RETURN TO FUNCTIONAL LIFE TOOK DECADES.
I USED TO GO FOR LONG PERIODS WITHOUT DOING ANYTHING, BUT NOW I PLAY EVERY DAY.
FINISHING THE ALBUM "SMILE" WAS MY BIGGEST ACCOMPLISHMENT ...EVER.
WILSON CONTINUES TO BOTH RECORD AND PERFORM. ONE OF THE FEW TRUE GENIUSES OF POPULAR MUSIC.

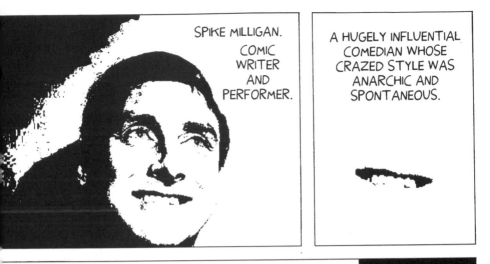

SPIKE MILLIGAN. COMIC WRITER AND PERFORMER.

A HUGELY INFLUENTIAL COMEDIAN WHOSE CRAZED STYLE WAS ANARCHIC AND SPONTANEOUS.

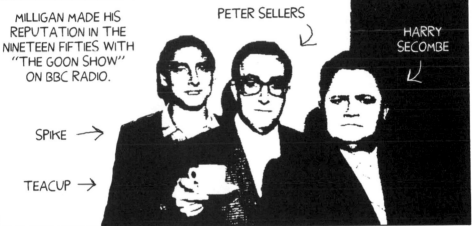

MILLIGAN MADE HIS REPUTATION IN THE NINETEEN FIFTIES WITH "THE GOON SHOW" ON BBC RADIO.

PETER SELLERS

HARRY SECOMBE

SPIKE →

TEACUP →

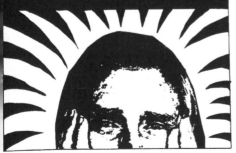

HE WROTE THE MAJORITY OF THE PROGRAMS AND PLAYED MANY OF THE PARTS.

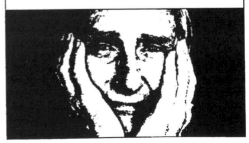

A HUGE WORKLOAD FOR MILLIGAN, WHICH LEFT HIM IN A STATE OF COMPLETE EMOTIONAL AND MENTAL COLLAPSE.

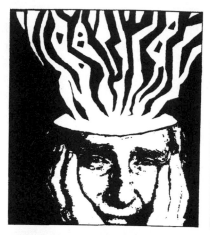

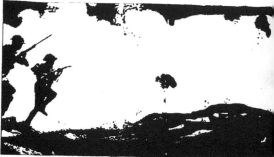

WOUNDED AND SHELLSHOCKED DURING THE SECOND WORLD WAR,

MILLIGAN SUFFERED BIPOLAR DISORDER THROUGHOUT HIS LIFE.

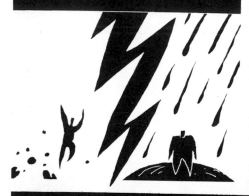

HE HAD AT LEAST TEN PSYCHIATRIC BREAKDOWNS, SEVERAL LASTING OVER A YEAR.

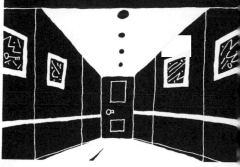

ELEVATED MOODS WOULD ALTERNATE WITH DEEP DEPRESSIONS.

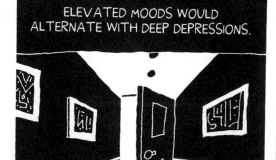

DID MILLIGAN'S ILLNESS UNLOCK A DOOR IN HIS MIND TO A WORLD OF COMEDY GENIUS?

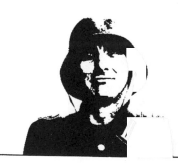

AN ELEVATED MOOD WILL BRING
WITH IT AN EXPLOSION OF ENERGY
AND FREE-FLOWING IDEAS.

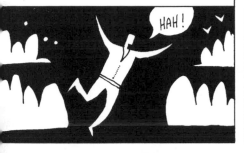

BUT THE INGENUITY AND ABILITY
TO THINK CREATIVELY HAS TO BE
THERE IN THE FIRST PLACE.

MENTAL ILLNESS WILL TEND TO
HINDER THE CREATIVE PROCESS
AS MUCH AS HELP IT.

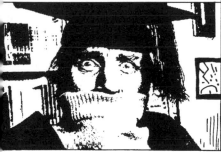

IT IS DESPITE MILLIGAN'S ILLNESS
THAT HE WAS A SUCCESSFUL AUTHOR,
NOT BECAUSE OF IT.

A TROUBLED, GIFTED MAN
WITH A UNIQUE WORLDVIEW.

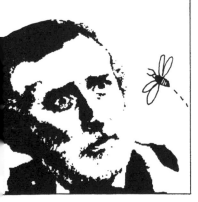

DO YOU FIND YOURSELF
LOOKING BACK ON YOUR
CHILDHOOD?

NO.
IT HURTS
MY NECK.

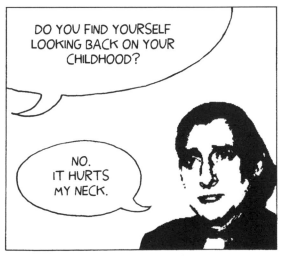

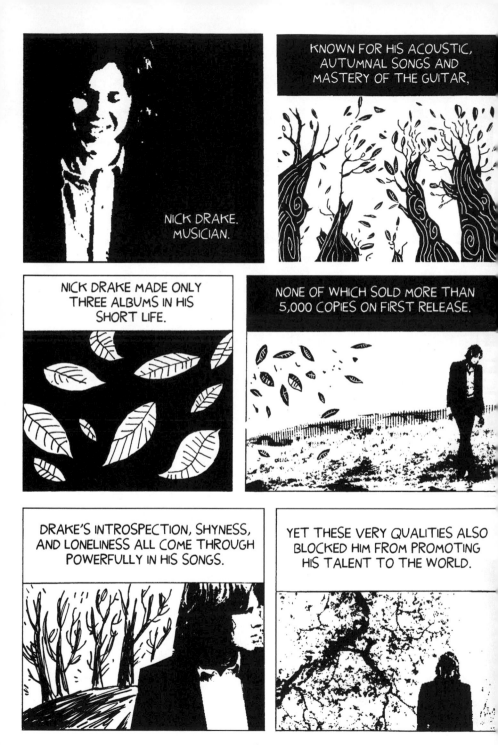

NICK DRAKE.
MUSICIAN.

KNOWN FOR HIS ACOUSTIC, AUTUMNAL SONGS AND MASTERY OF THE GUITAR,

NICK DRAKE MADE ONLY THREE ALBUMS IN HIS SHORT LIFE.

NONE OF WHICH SOLD MORE THAN 5,000 COPIES ON FIRST RELEASE.

DRAKE'S INTROSPECTION, SHYNESS, AND LONELINESS ALL COME THROUGH POWERFULLY IN HIS SONGS.

YET THESE VERY QUALITIES ALSO BLOCKED HIM FROM PROMOTING HIS TALENT TO THE WORLD.

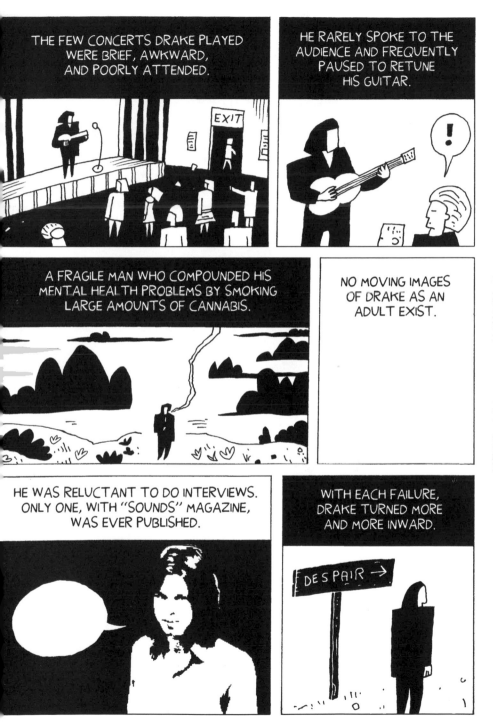

THE FEW CONCERTS DRAKE PLAYED WERE BRIEF, AWKWARD, AND POORLY ATTENDED.

HE RARELY SPOKE TO THE AUDIENCE AND FREQUENTLY PAUSED TO RETUNE HIS GUITAR.

A FRAGILE MAN WHO COMPOUNDED HIS MENTAL HEALTH PROBLEMS BY SMOKING LARGE AMOUNTS OF CANNABIS.

NO MOVING IMAGES OF DRAKE AS AN ADULT EXIST.

HE WAS RELUCTANT TO DO INTERVIEWS. ONLY ONE, WITH "SOUNDS" MAGAZINE, WAS EVER PUBLISHED.

WITH EACH FAILURE, DRAKE TURNED MORE AND MORE INWARD.

DESPAIR →

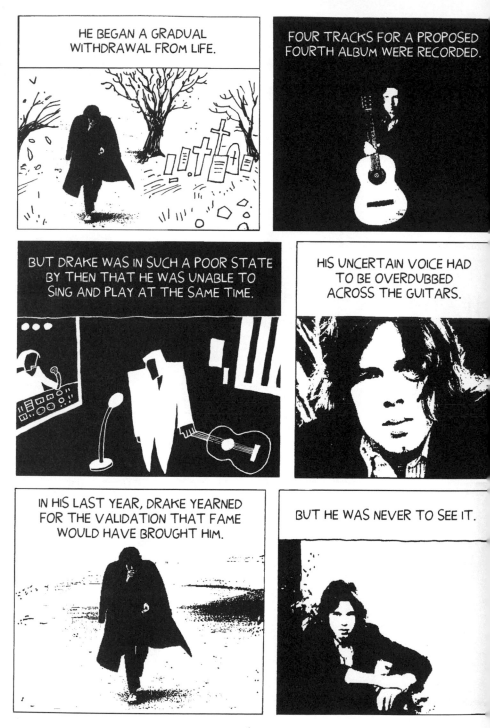

HE BEGAN A GRADUAL WITHDRAWAL FROM LIFE.

FOUR TRACKS FOR A PROPOSED FOURTH ALBUM WERE RECORDED.

BUT DRAKE WAS IN SUCH A POOR STATE BY THEN THAT HE WAS UNABLE TO SING AND PLAY AT THE SAME TIME.

HIS UNCERTAIN VOICE HAD TO BE OVERDUBBED ACROSS THE GUITARS.

IN HIS LAST YEAR, DRAKE YEARNED FOR THE VALIDATION THAT FAME WOULD HAVE BROUGHT HIM.

BUT HE WAS NEVER TO SEE IT.

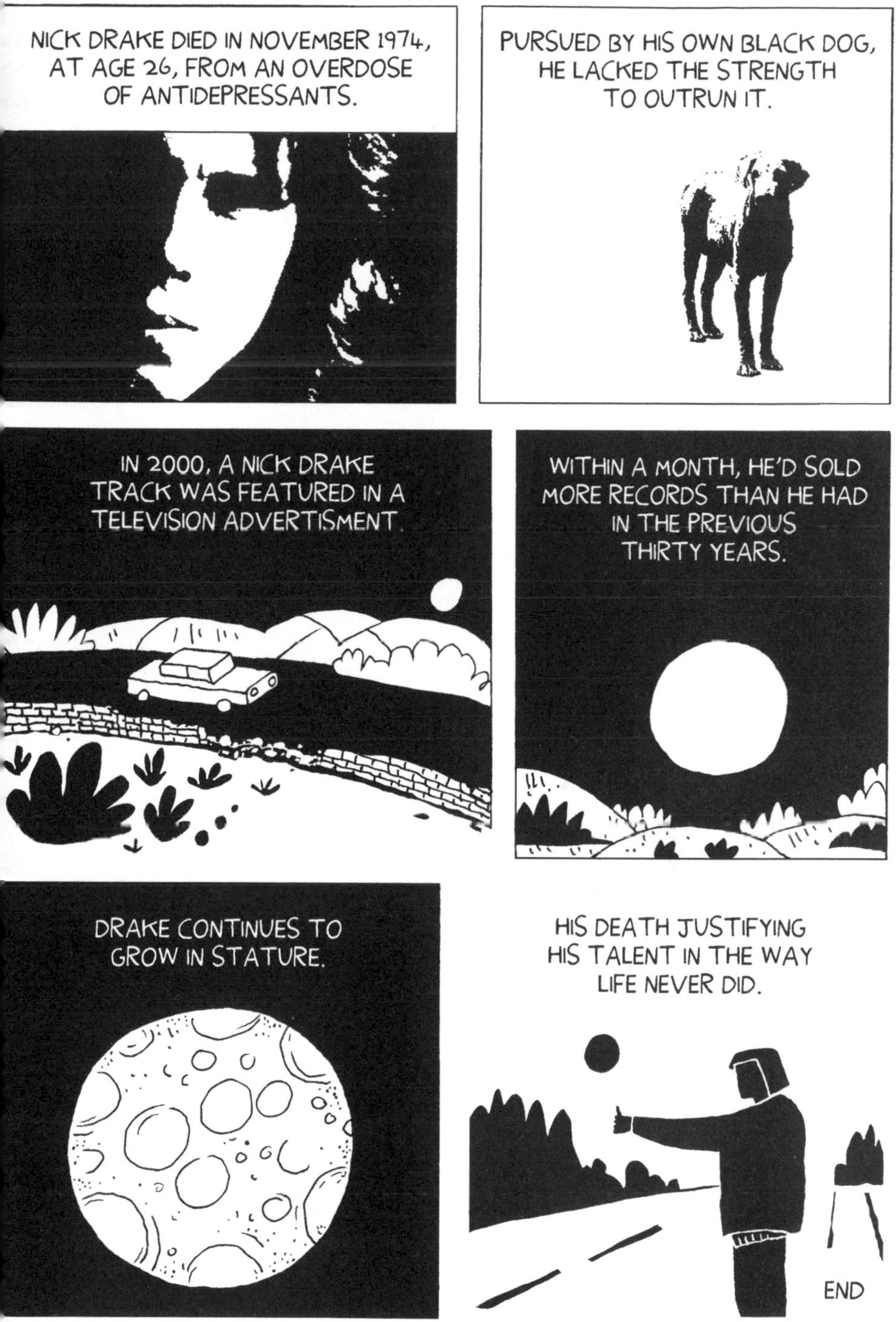

NICK DRAKE DIED IN NOVEMBER 1974, AT AGE 26, FROM AN OVERDOSE OF ANTIDEPRESSANTS.

PURSUED BY HIS OWN BLACK DOG, HE LACKED THE STRENGTH TO OUTRUN IT.

IN 2000, A NICK DRAKE TRACK WAS FEATURED IN A TELEVISION ADVERTISMENT.

WITHIN A MONTH, HE'D SOLD MORE RECORDS THAN HE HAD IN THE PREVIOUS THIRTY YEARS.

DRAKE CONTINUES TO GROW IN STATURE.

HIS DEATH JUSTIFYING HIS TALENT IN THE WAY LIFE NEVER DID.

END

65

BLOOD

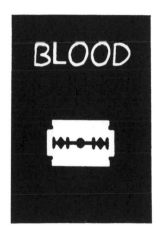

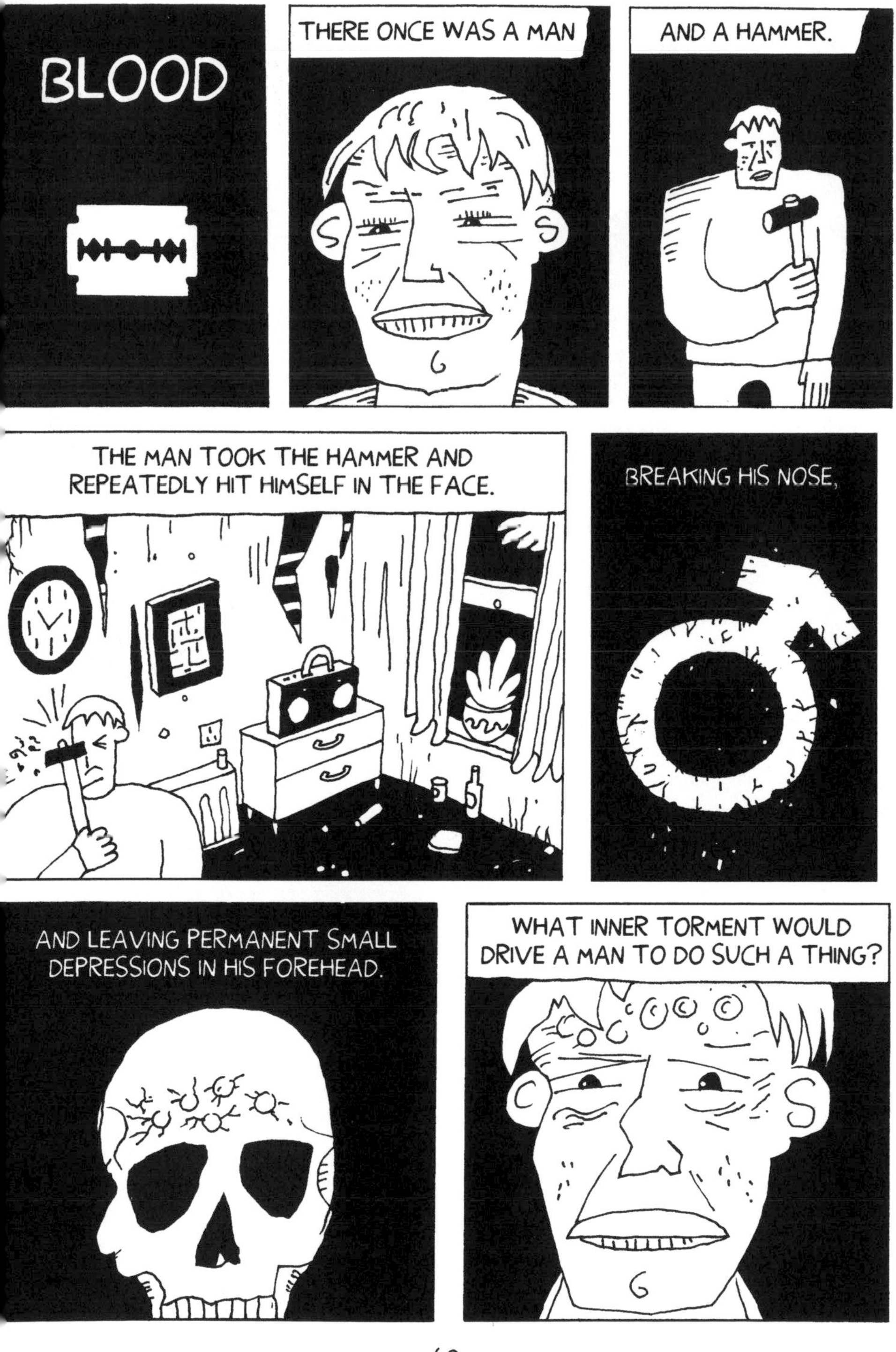
BLOOD
THERE ONCE WAS A MAN
AND A HAMMER.
THE MAN TOOK THE HAMMER AND REPEATEDLY HIT HIMSELF IN THE FACE.
BREAKING HIS NOSE,
AND LEAVING PERMANENT SMALL DEPRESSIONS IN HIS FOREHEAD.
WHAT INNER TORMENT WOULD DRIVE A MAN TO DO SUCH A THING?

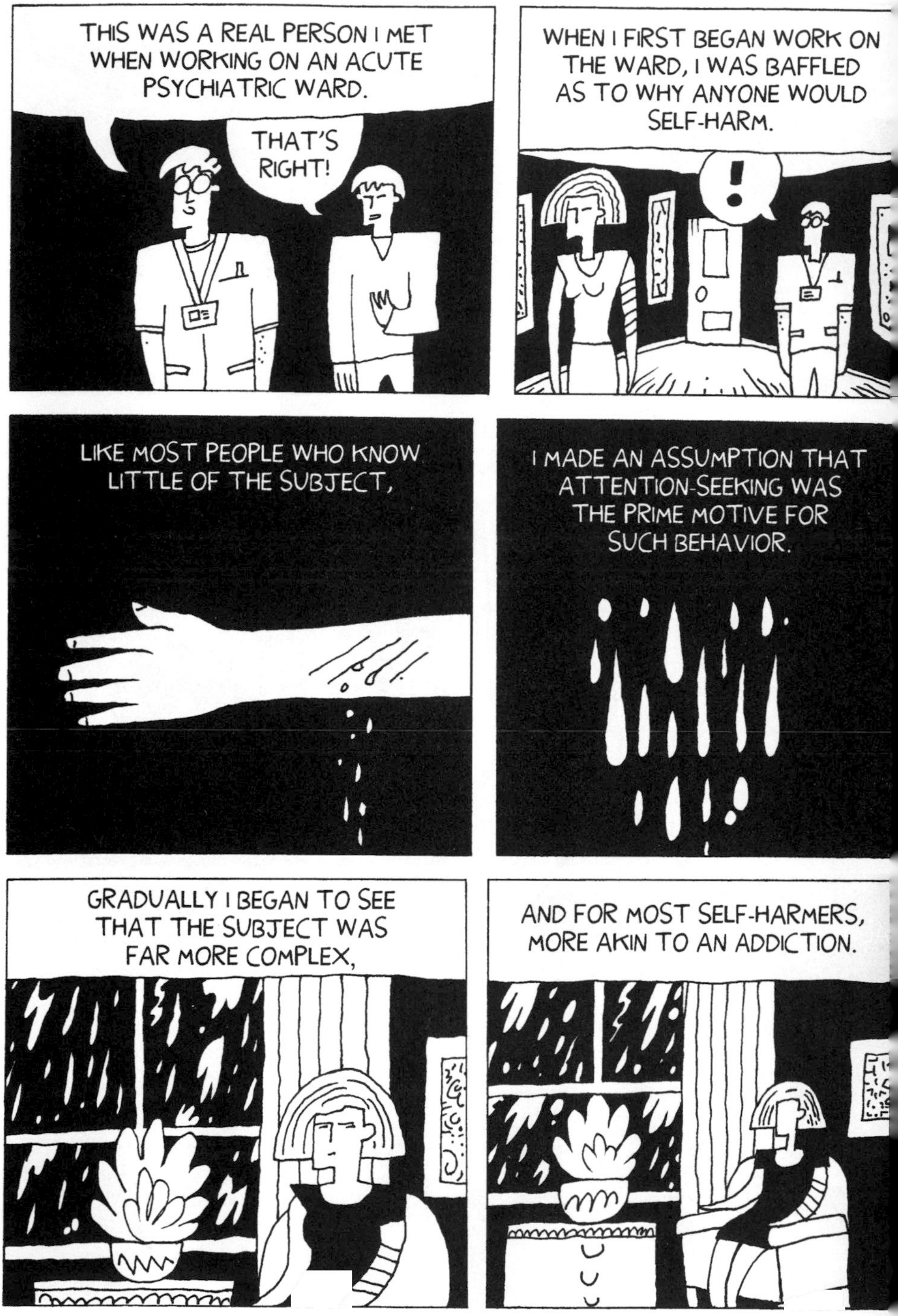
THIS WAS A REAL PERSON I MET WHEN WORKING ON AN ACUTE PSYCHIATRIC WARD.
THAT'S RIGHT!
WHEN I FIRST BEGAN WORK ON THE WARD, I WAS BAFFLED AS TO WHY ANYONE WOULD SELF-HARM.
!
LIKE MOST PEOPLE WHO KNOW LITTLE OF THE SUBJECT,
I MADE AN ASSUMPTION THAT ATTENTION-SEEKING WAS THE PRIME MOTIVE FOR SUCH BEHAVIOR.
GRADUALLY I BEGAN TO SEE THAT THE SUBJECT WAS FAR MORE COMPLEX,
AND FOR MOST SELF-HARMERS, MORE AKIN TO AN ADDICTION.

AN ADDICTION WITH BOTH PSYCHOLOGICAL AND PHYSICAL ASPECTS TO IT.

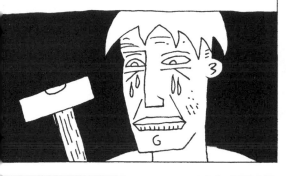

SELF-HARMING IS BEST UNDERSTOOD AS A COPING MECHANISM.

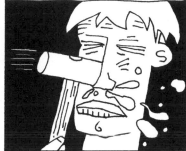

PHYSICAL INJURY RELEASES BETA ENDORPHINS IN THE BRAIN THAT CAN ACT AS PAINKILLERS,

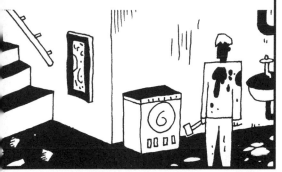

AS WELL AS INDUCING PLEASANT FEELINGS AND REDUCING TENSION,

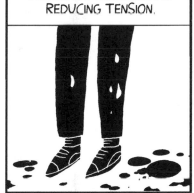

PAIN PROVIDES TEMPORARY RELIEF AGAINST UNBEARABLE EMOTIONAL DISTRESS.

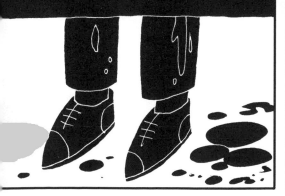

SUFFERERS EXPERIENCE A TURMOIL OF DEPRESSION, ANXIETY, AND SELF-LOATHING.

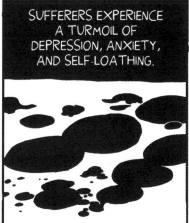

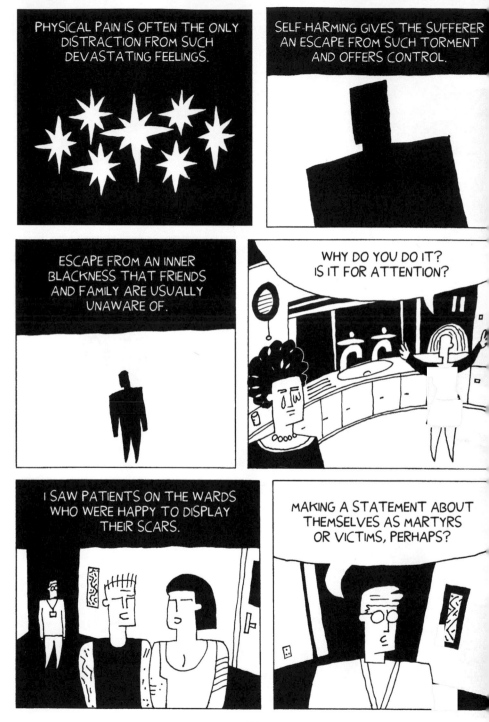

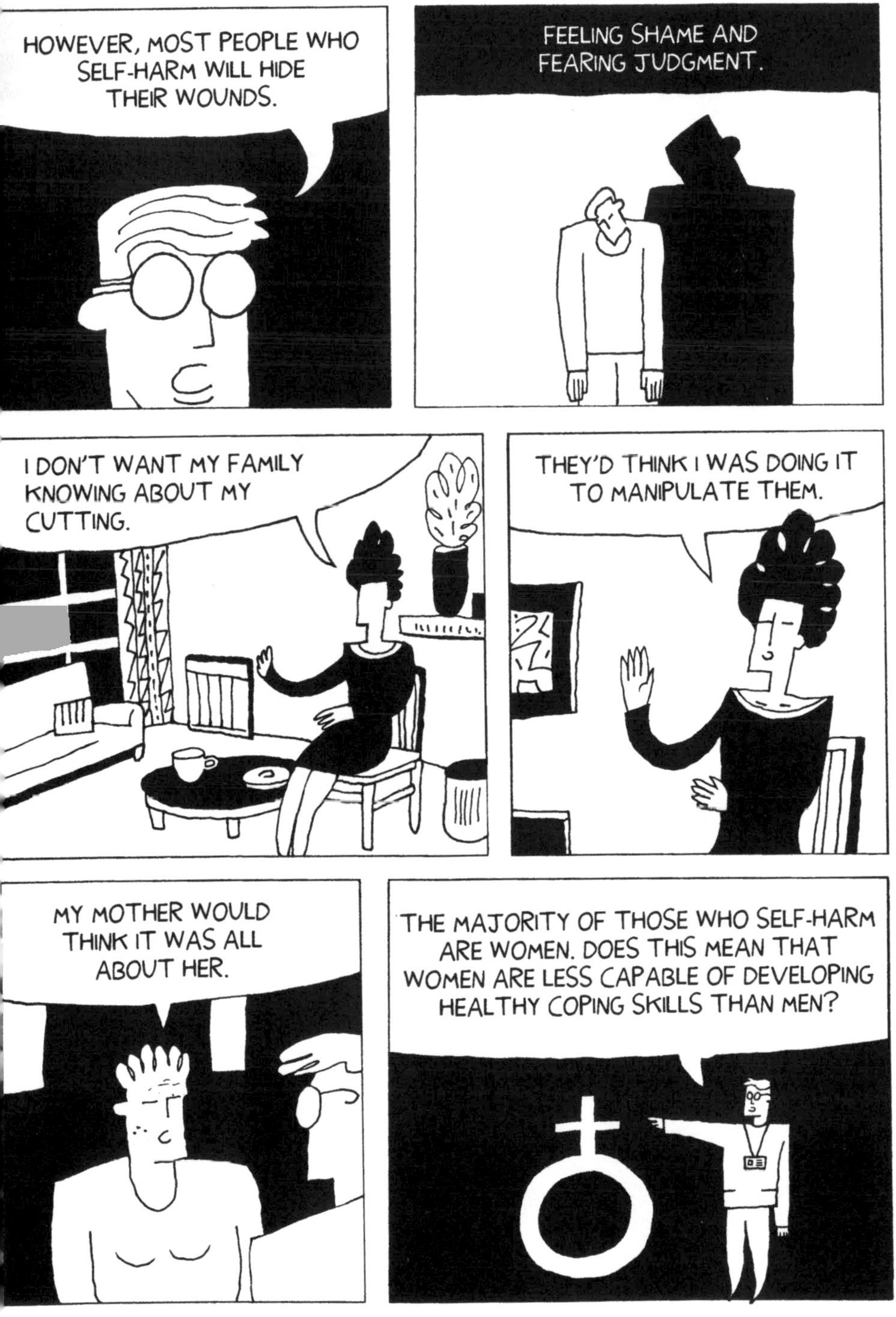
HOWEVER, MOST PEOPLE WHO SELF-HARM WILL HIDE THEIR WOUNDS.
FEELING SHAME AND FEARING JUDGMENT.
I DON'T WANT MY FAMILY KNOWING ABOUT MY CUTTING.
THEY'D THINK I WAS DOING IT TO MANIPULATE THEM.
MY MOTHER WOULD THINK IT WAS ALL ABOUT HER.
THE MAJORITY OF THOSE WHO SELF-HARM ARE WOMEN. DOES THIS MEAN THAT WOMEN ARE LESS CAPABLE OF DEVELOPING HEALTHY COPING SKILLS THAN MEN?

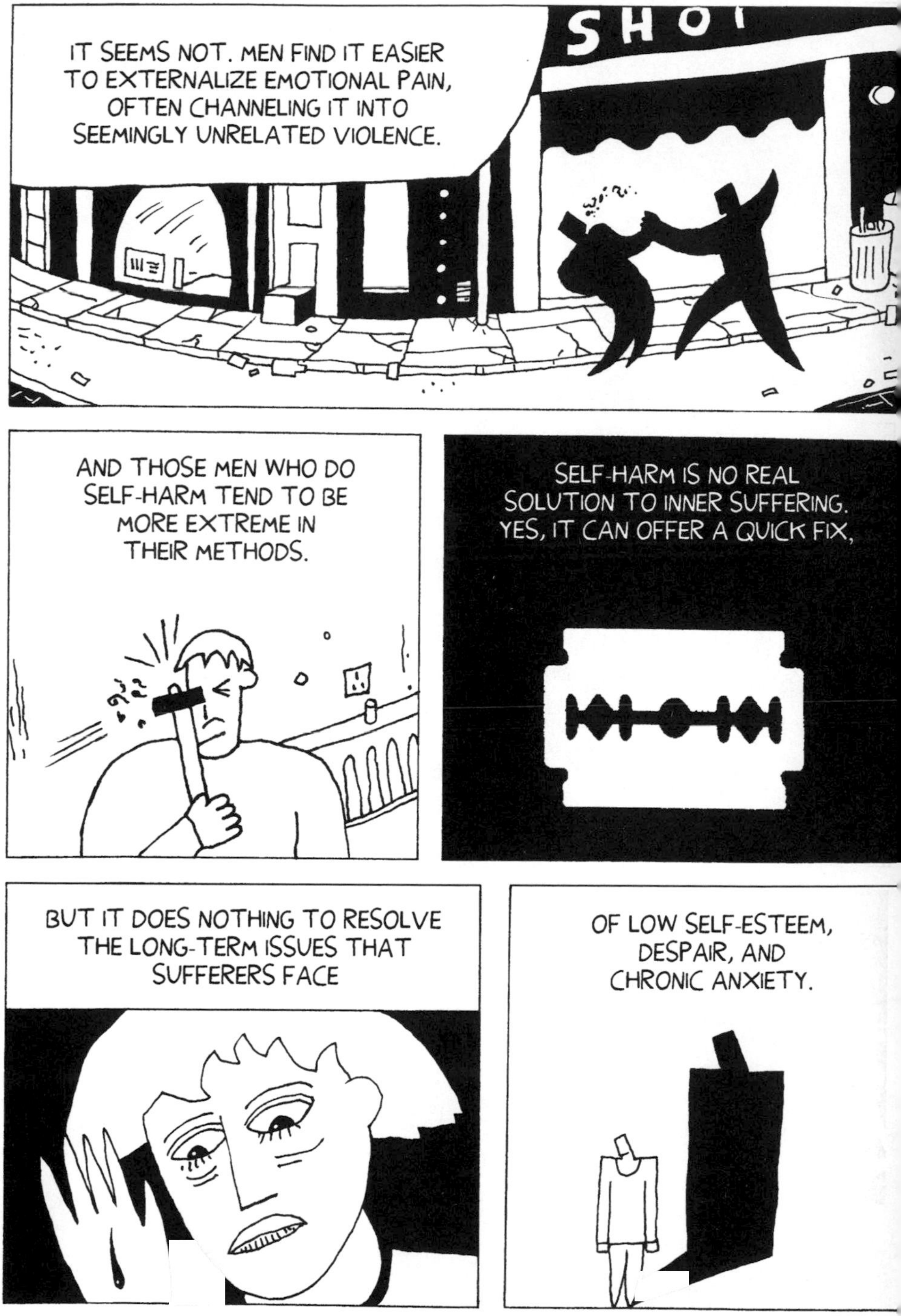
IT SEEMS NOT. MEN FIND IT EASIER TO EXTERNALIZE EMOTIONAL PAIN, OFTEN CHANNELING IT INTO SEEMINGLY UNRELATED VIOLENCE.
AND THOSE MEN WHO DO SELF-HARM TEND TO BE MORE EXTREME IN THEIR METHODS.
SELF-HARM IS NO REAL SOLUTION TO INNER SUFFERING. YES, IT CAN OFFER A QUICK FIX,
BUT IT DOES NOTHING TO RESOLVE THE LONG-TERM ISSUES THAT SUFFERERS FACE
OF LOW SELF-ESTEEM, DESPAIR, AND CHRONIC ANXIETY.

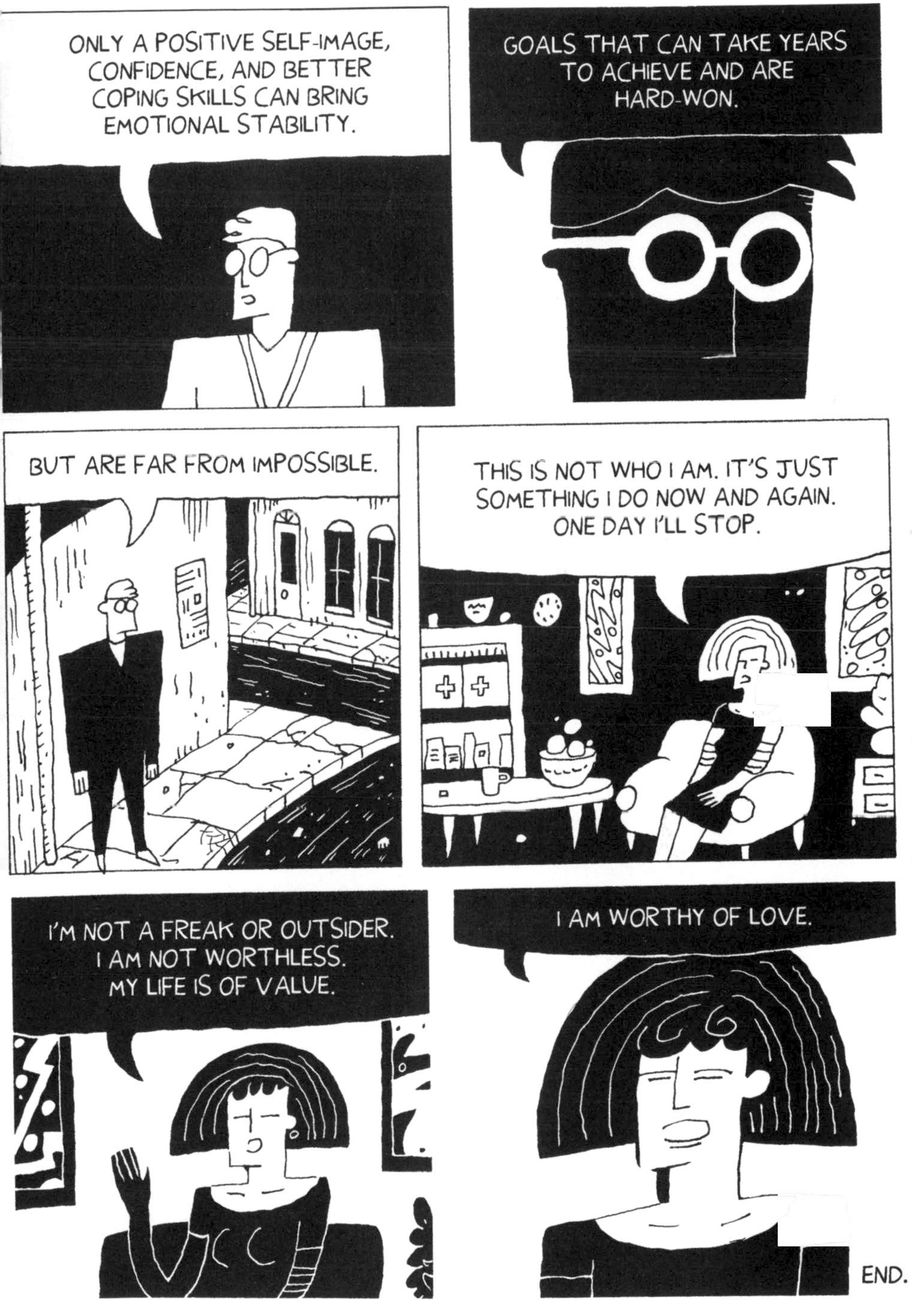
ONLY A POSITIVE SELF-IMAGE, CONFIDENCE, AND BETTER COPING SKILLS CAN BRING EMOTIONAL STABILITY.
GOALS THAT CAN TAKE YEARS TO ACHIEVE AND ARE HARD-WON.
BUT ARE FAR FROM IMPOSSIBLE.
THIS IS NOT WHO I AM. IT'S JUST SOMETHING I DO NOW AND AGAIN. ONE DAY I'LL STOP.
I'M NOT A FREAK OR OUTSIDER. I AM NOT WORTHLESS. MY LIFE IS OF VALUE.
I AM WORTHY OF LOVE.
END.

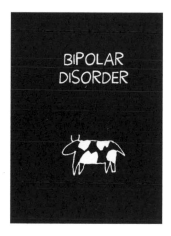

BIPOLAR
DISORDER

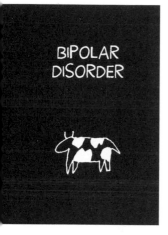

BIPOLAR
DISORDER

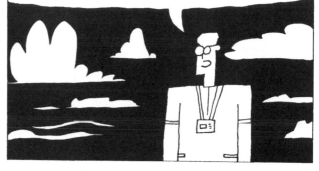

A STAFF NURSE WHO I WORKED WITH ON A PSYCHIATRIC WARD BELIEVED THAT YOU COULD ALWAYS TELL WHO THE BIPOLAR PATIENTS WERE

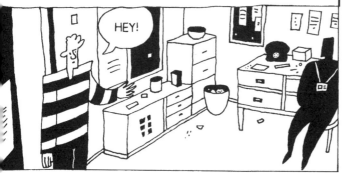

BECAUSE THEY WERE THE PATIENTS WHO WOULD BE UNABLE TO WALK PAST THE OFFICE WITHOUT COMING IN TO EXPLAIN WHATEVER WAS ON THEIR MIND,

HEY!

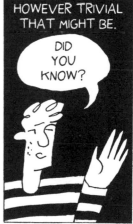

HOWEVER TRIVIAL THAT MIGHT BE.

DID YOU KNOW?

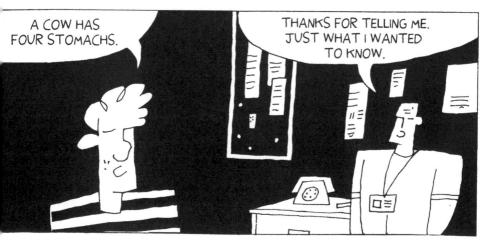

A COW HAS FOUR STOMACHS.

THANKS FOR TELLING ME. JUST WHAT I WANTED TO KNOW.

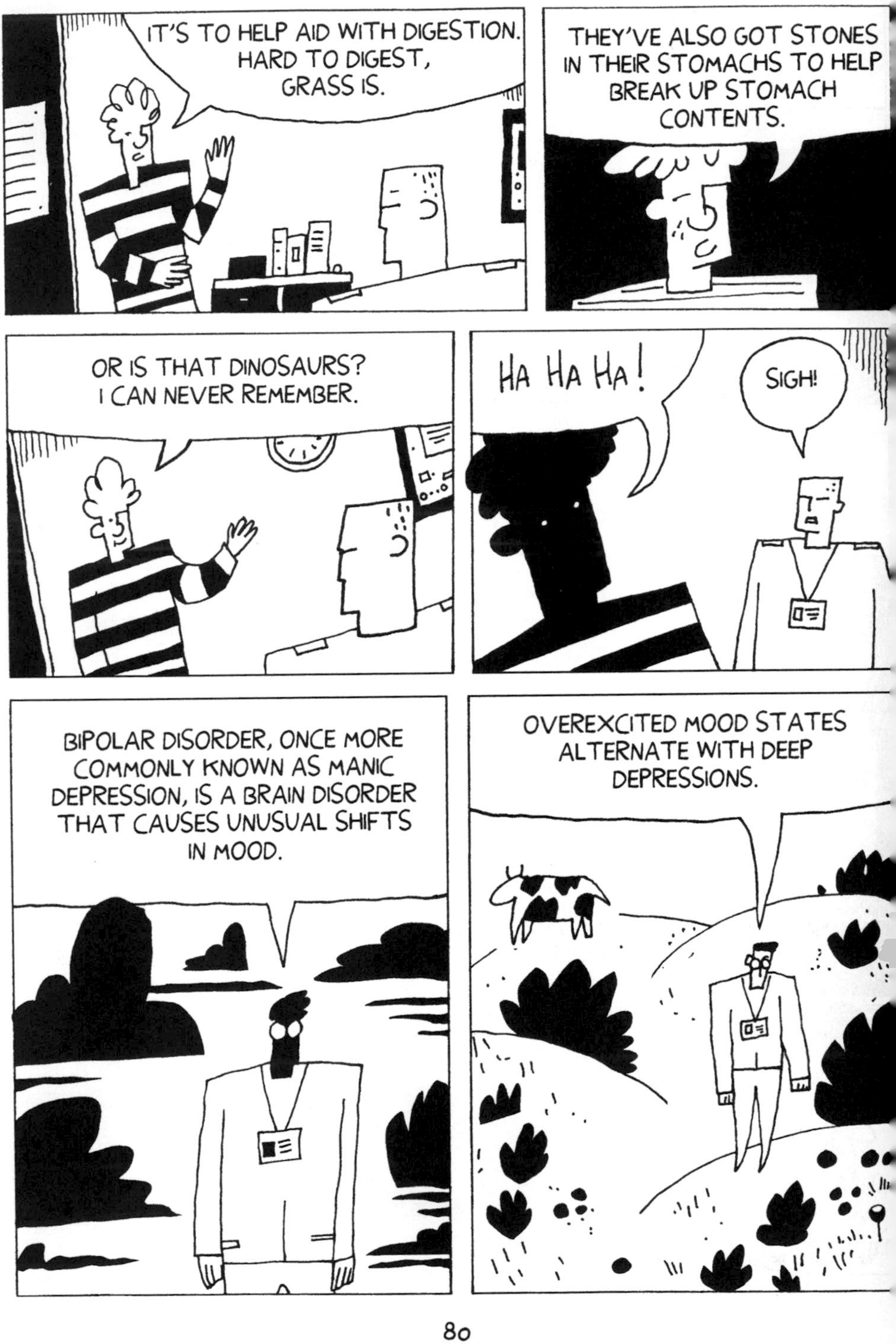
IT'S TO HELP AID WITH DIGESTION. HARD TO DIGEST, GRASS IS.
THEY'VE ALSO GOT STONES IN THEIR STOMACHS TO HELP BREAK UP STOMACH CONTENTS.
OR IS THAT DINOSAURS? I CAN NEVER REMEMBER.
HA HA HA!
SIGH!
BIPOLAR DISORDER, ONCE MORE COMMONLY KNOWN AS MANIC DEPRESSION, IS A BRAIN DISORDER THAT CAUSES UNUSUAL SHIFTS IN MOOD.
OVEREXCITED MOOD STATES ALTERNATE WITH DEEP DEPRESSIONS.

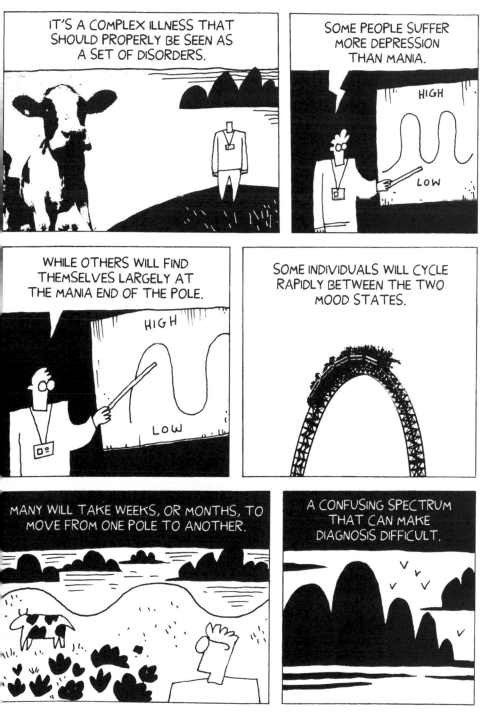

81

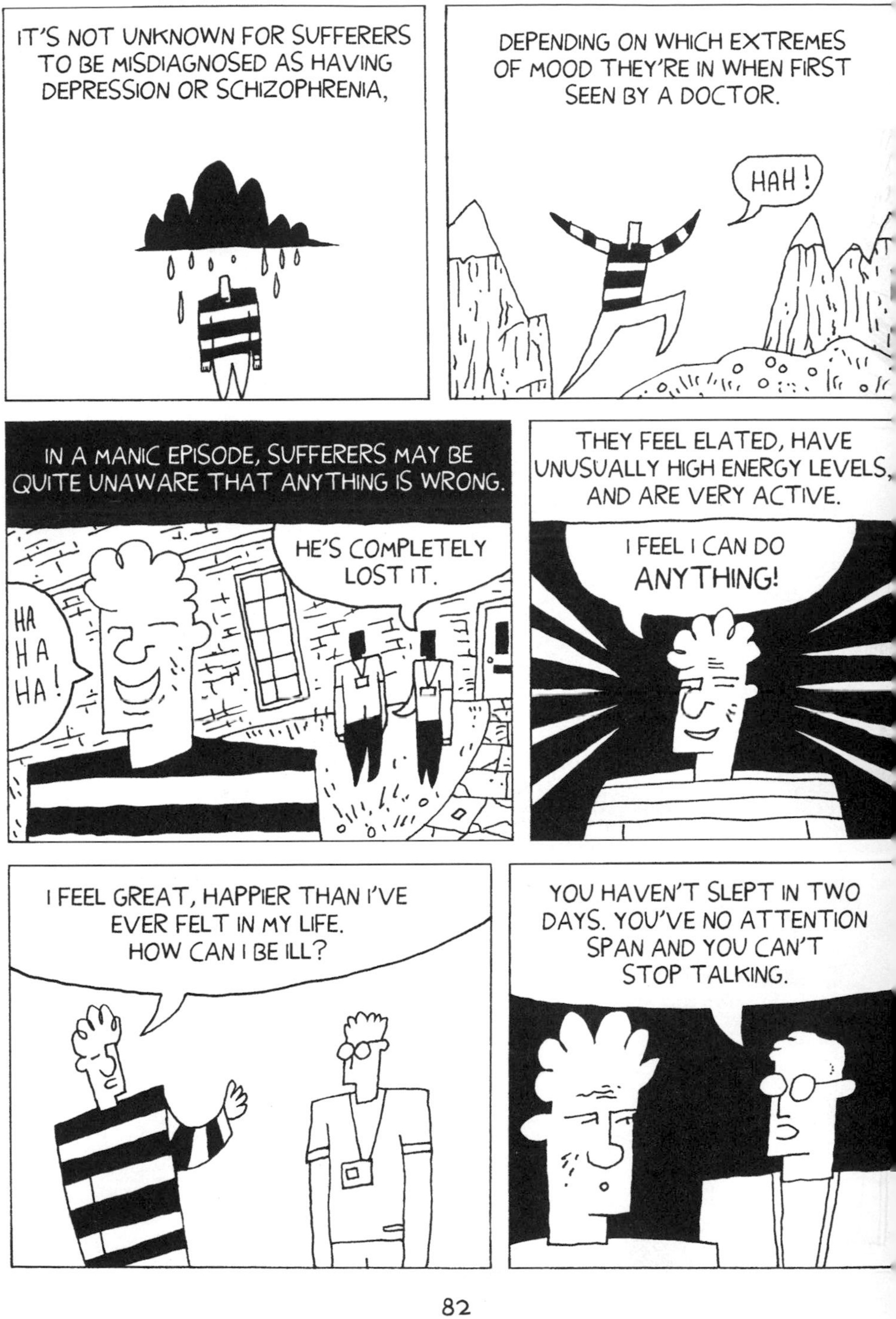
IT'S NOT UNKNOWN FOR SUFFERERS TO BE MISDIAGNOSED AS HAVING DEPRESSION OR SCHIZOPHRENIA,
DEPENDING ON WHICH EXTREMES OF MOOD THEY'RE IN WHEN FIRST SEEN BY A DOCTOR.
HAH!
IN A MANIC EPISODE, SUFFERERS MAY BE QUITE UNAWARE THAT ANYTHING IS WRONG.
HE'S COMPLETELY LOST IT.
HA HA HA!
THEY FEEL ELATED, HAVE UNUSUALLY HIGH ENERGY LEVELS, AND ARE VERY ACTIVE.
I FEEL I CAN DO ANYTHING!
I FEEL GREAT, HAPPIER THAN I'VE EVER FELT IN MY LIFE. HOW CAN I BE ILL?
YOU HAVEN'T SLEPT IN TWO DAYS. YOU'VE NO ATTENTION SPAN AND YOU CAN'T STOP TALKING.

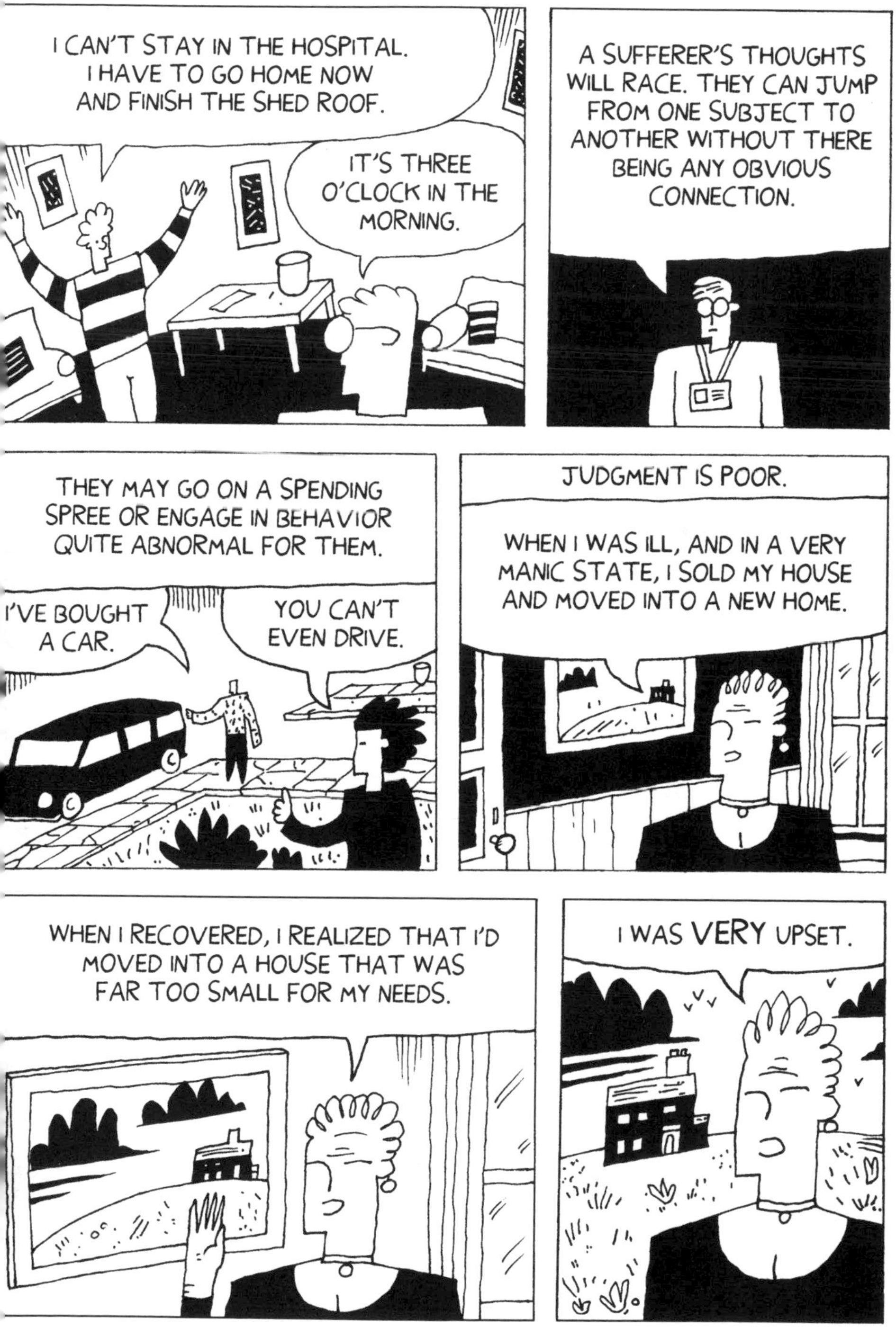
I CAN'T STAY IN THE HOSPITAL. I HAVE TO GO HOME NOW AND FINISH THE SHED ROOF.
IT'S THREE O'CLOCK IN THE MORNING.
A SUFFERER'S THOUGHTS WILL RACE. THEY CAN JUMP FROM ONE SUBJECT TO ANOTHER WITHOUT THERE BEING ANY OBVIOUS CONNECTION.
THEY MAY GO ON A SPENDING SPREE OR ENGAGE IN BEHAVIOR QUITE ABNORMAL FOR THEM.
I'VE BOUGHT A CAR.
YOU CAN'T EVEN DRIVE.
JUDGMENT IS POOR.
WHEN I WAS ILL, AND IN A VERY MANIC STATE, I SOLD MY HOUSE AND MOVED INTO A NEW HOME.
WHEN I RECOVERED, I REALIZED THAT I'D MOVED INTO A HOUSE THAT WAS FAR TOO SMALL FOR MY NEEDS.
I WAS VERY UPSET.

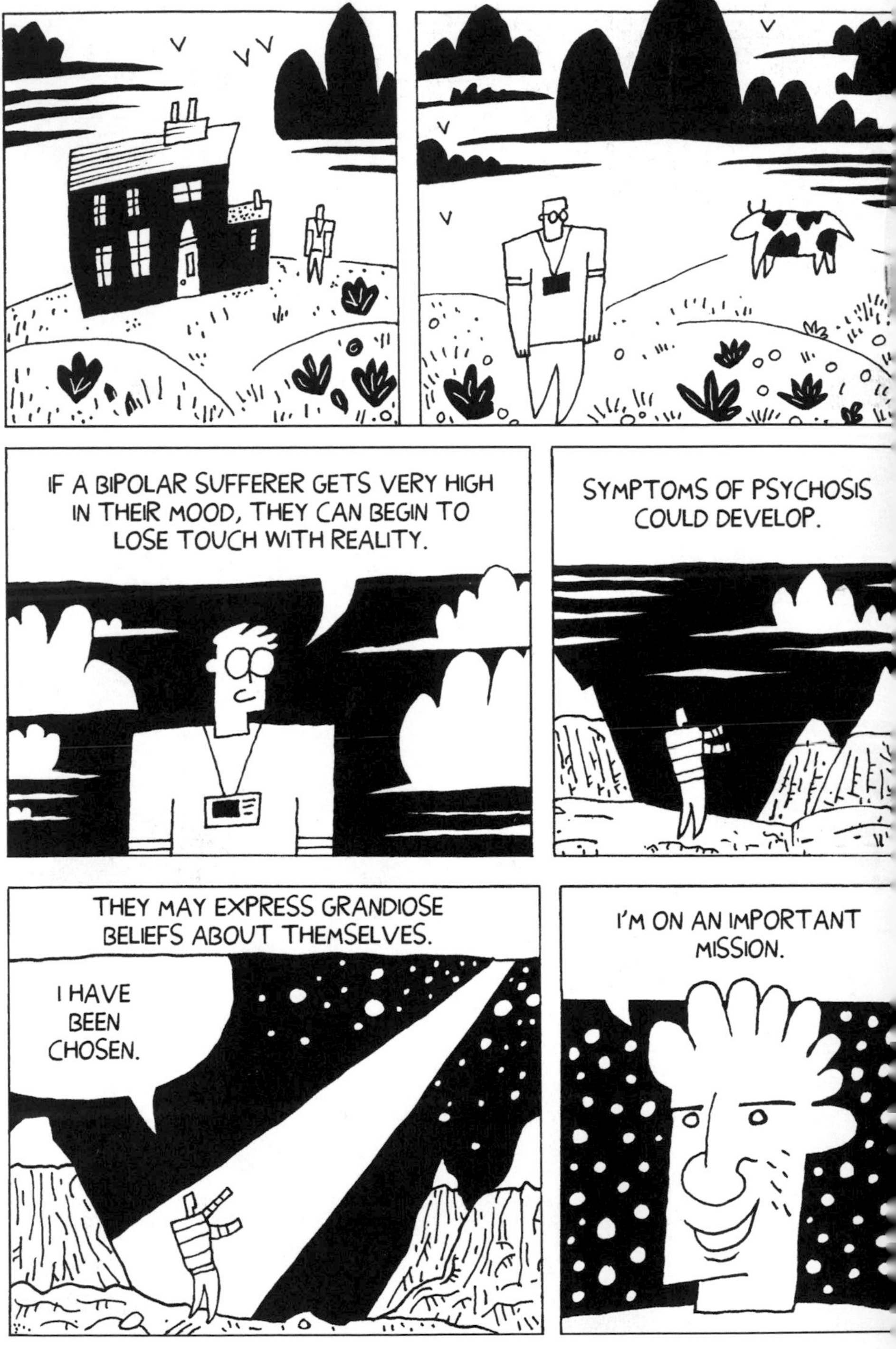
IF A BIPOLAR SUFFERER GETS VERY HIGH IN THEIR MOOD, THEY CAN BEGIN TO LOSE TOUCH WITH REALITY.
SYMPTOMS OF PSYCHOSIS COULD DEVELOP.
THEY MAY EXPRESS GRANDIOSE BELIEFS ABOUT THEMSELVES.
I HAVE BEEN CHOSEN.
I'M ON AN IMPORTANT MISSION.

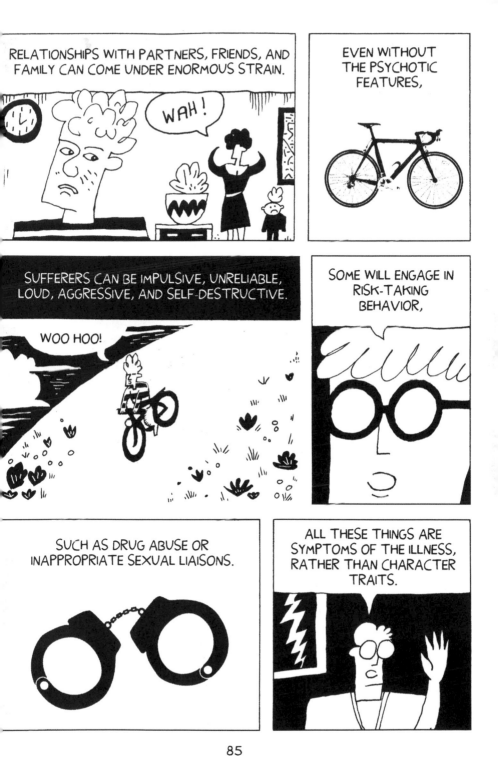

RELATIONSHIPS WITH PARTNERS, FRIENDS, AND FAMILY CAN COME UNDER ENORMOUS STRAIN.

WAH!

EVEN WITHOUT THE PSYCHOTIC FEATURES,

SUFFERERS CAN BE IMPULSIVE, UNRELIABLE, LOUD, AGGRESSIVE, AND SELF-DESTRUCTIVE.

WOO HOO!

SOME WILL ENGAGE IN RISK-TAKING BEHAVIOR,

SUCH AS DRUG ABUSE OR INAPPROPRIATE SEXUAL LIAISONS.

ALL THESE THINGS ARE SYMPTOMS OF THE ILLNESS, RATHER THAN CHARACTER TRAITS.

85

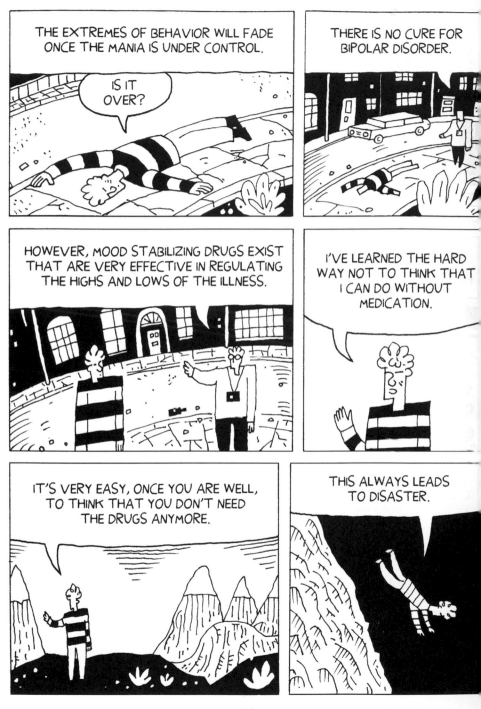

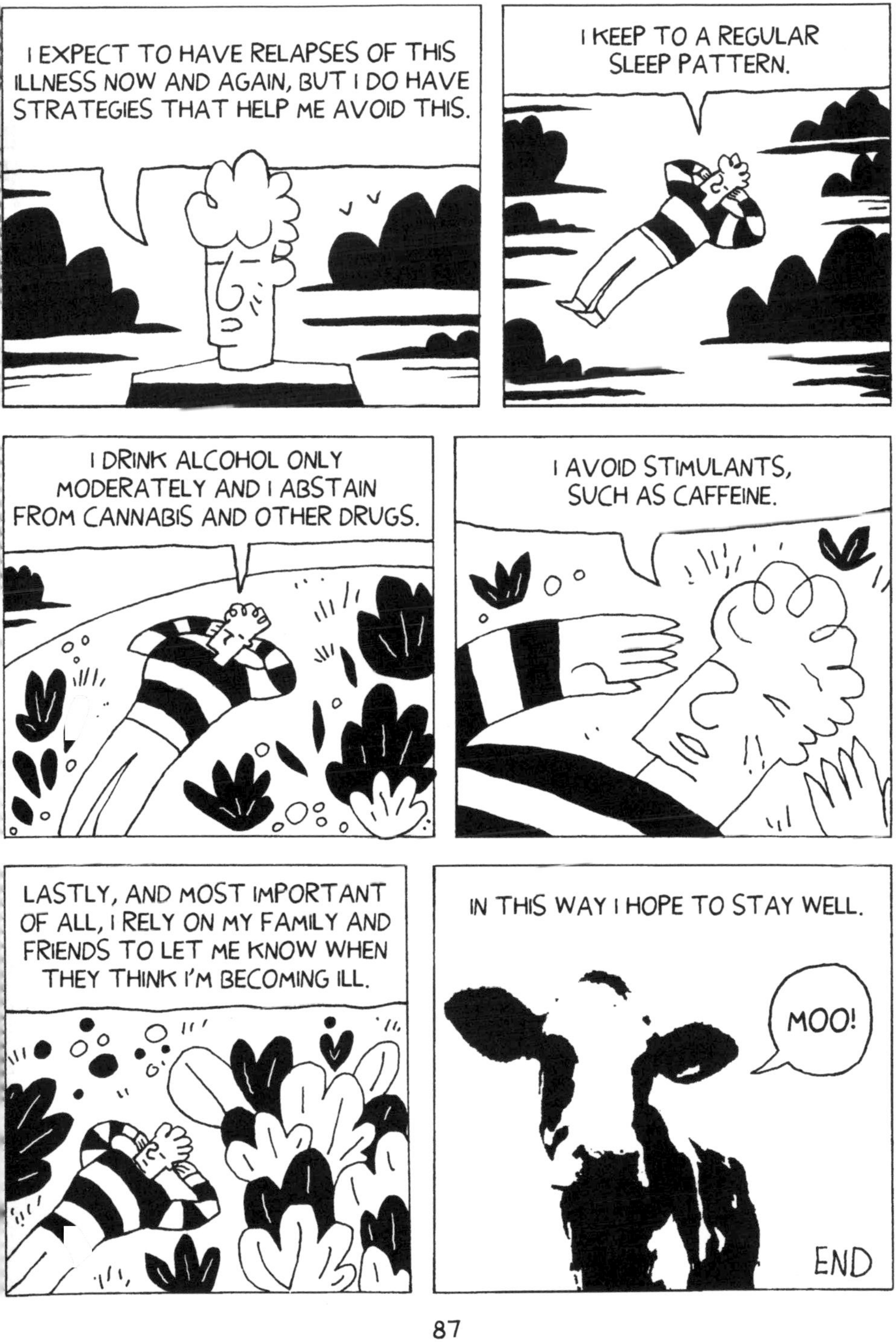
I EXPECT TO HAVE RELAPSES OF THIS ILLNESS NOW AND AGAIN, BUT I DO HAVE STRATEGIES THAT HELP ME AVOID THIS.
I KEEP TO A REGULAR SLEEP PATTERN.
I DRINK ALCOHOL ONLY MODERATELY AND I ABSTAIN FROM CANNABIS AND OTHER DRUGS.
I AVOID STIMULANTS, SUCH AS CAFFEINE.
LASTLY, AND MOST IMPORTANT OF ALL, I RELY ON MY FAMILY AND FRIENDS TO LET ME KNOW WHEN THEY THINK I'M BECOMING ILL.
IN THIS WAY I HOPE TO STAY WELL.
MOO!
END

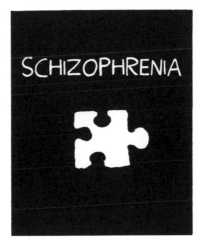

SCHIZOPHRENIA

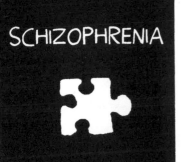

SCHIZOPHRENIA

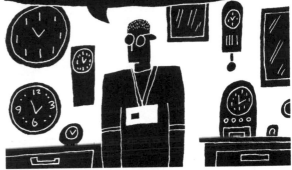

SUFFERERS OF SCHIZOPHRENIA DON'T HAVE MULTIPLE PERSONALITY DISORDER.

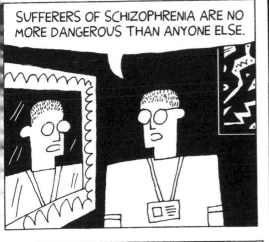

SUFFERERS OF SCHIZOPHRENIA ARE NO MORE DANGEROUS THAN ANYONE ELSE.

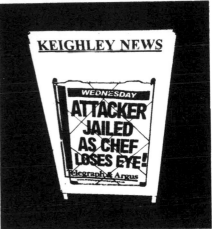

MURDERS COMMITTED BY PEOPLE WITH THIS ILLNESS ARE QUITE RARE, DESPITE MEDIA SENSATIONALISM.

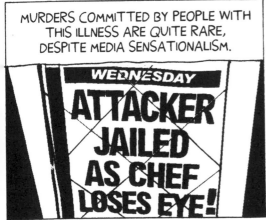

CRIMES INVOLVING THE MENTALLY ILL TEND TO GET PUBLICITY OUT OF PROPORTION TO THEIR FREQUENCY.

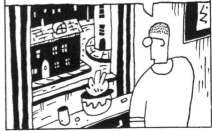

91

WHY IS THIS?

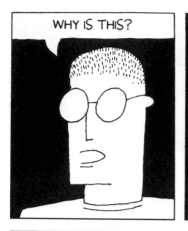

IT'S BECAUSE THERE'S MUCH FEAR AND IGNORANCE IN THE GENERAL POPULATION ON THE SUBJECT OF SCHIZOPHRENIA.

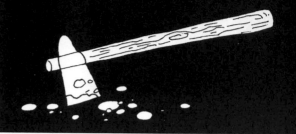

THESE FEW INCIDENTS MAKE FOR EASY AND LAZY NEWS STORIES.

NEWS

MAD KILLER!

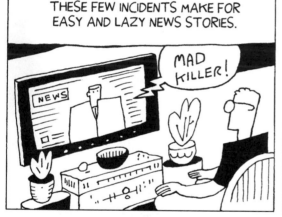

SCHIZOPHRENIA IS A BRAIN DISORDER THAT CREATES DISTORTIONS IN PERCEPTIONS AND THINKING.

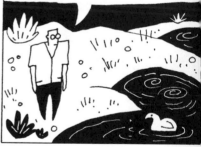

THE SUFFERER'S REALITY CAN BE TWISTED AND DISTORTED IN BIZARRE WAYS.

I DON'T LIKE TO GO OUT MUCH AS PEOPLE READ MY MIND.

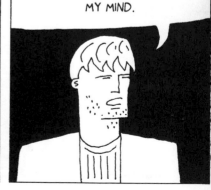

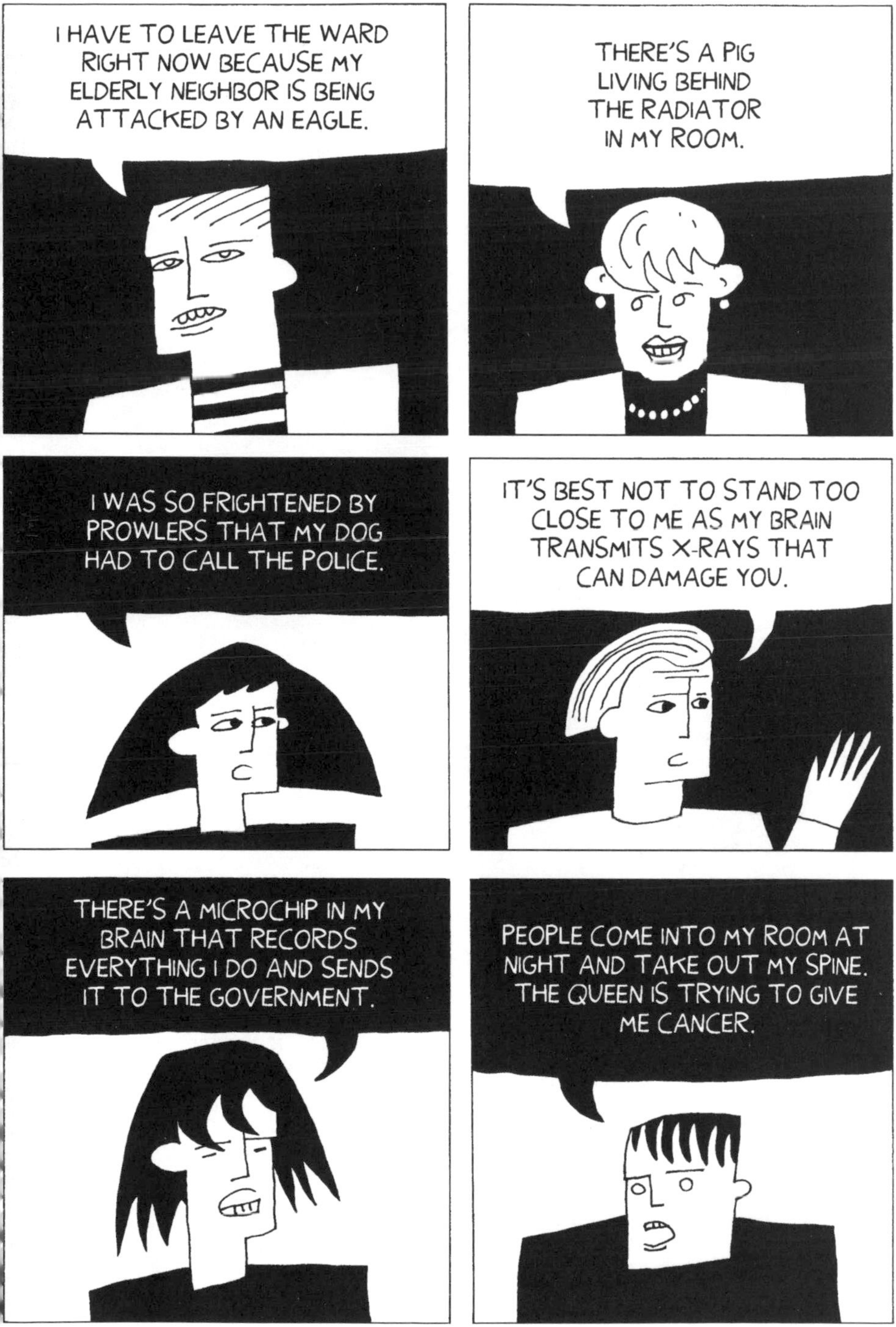
I HAVE TO LEAVE THE WARD RIGHT NOW BECAUSE MY ELDERLY NEIGHBOR IS BEING ATTACKED BY AN EAGLE.
THERE'S A PIG LIVING BEHIND THE RADIATOR IN MY ROOM.
I WAS SO FRIGHTENED BY PROWLERS THAT MY DOG HAD TO CALL THE POLICE.
IT'S BEST NOT TO STAND TOO CLOSE TO ME AS MY BRAIN TRANSMITS X-RAYS THAT CAN DAMAGE YOU.
THERE'S A MICROCHIP IN MY BRAIN THAT RECORDS EVERYTHING I DO AND SENDS IT TO THE GOVERNMENT.
PEOPLE COME INTO MY ROOM AT NIGHT AND TAKE OUT MY SPINE. THE QUEEN IS TRYING TO GIVE ME CANCER.

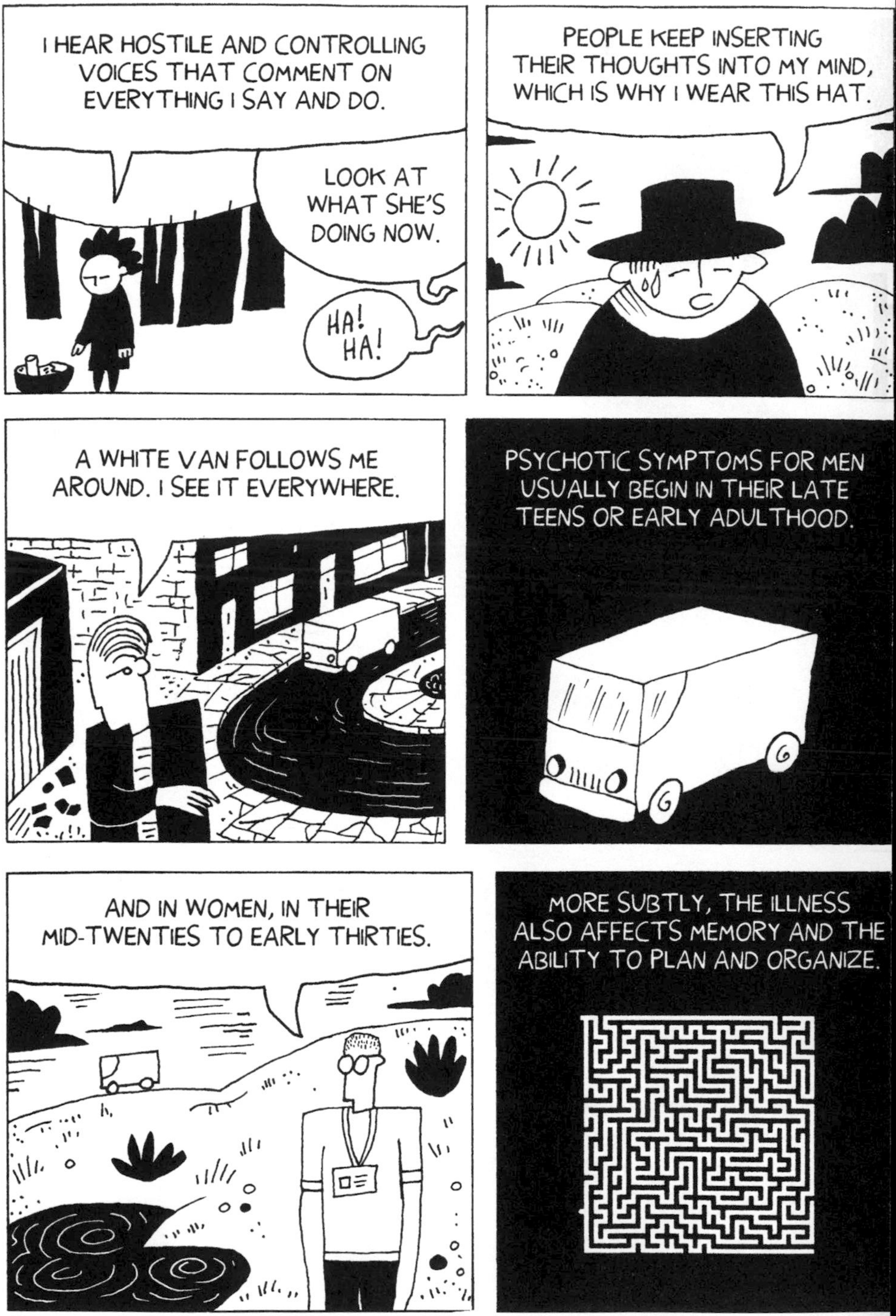

I HEAR HOSTILE AND CONTROLLING VOICES THAT COMMENT ON EVERYTHING I SAY AND DO.
LOOK AT WHAT SHE'S DOING NOW.
HA! HA!
PEOPLE KEEP INSERTING THEIR THOUGHTS INTO MY MIND, WHICH IS WHY I WEAR THIS HAT.
A WHITE VAN FOLLOWS ME AROUND. I SEE IT EVERYWHERE.
PSYCHOTIC SYMPTOMS FOR MEN USUALLY BEGIN IN THEIR LATE TEENS OR EARLY ADULTHOOD.
AND IN WOMEN, IN THEIR MID-TWENTIES TO EARLY THIRTIES.
MORE SUBTLY, THE ILLNESS ALSO AFFECTS MEMORY AND THE ABILITY TO PLAN AND ORGANIZE.

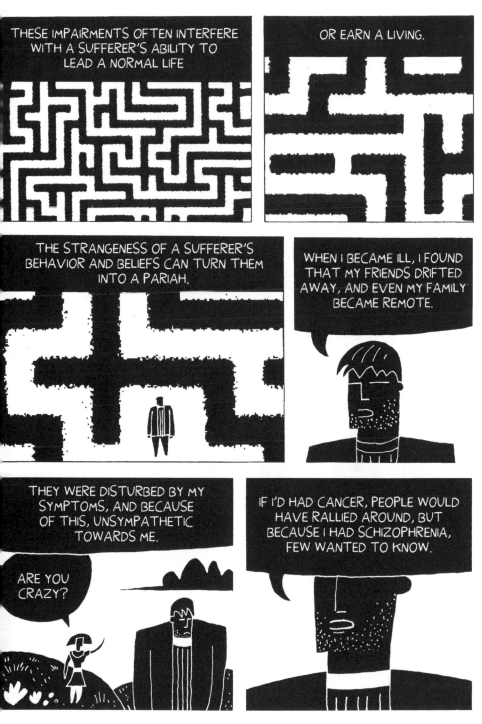

95

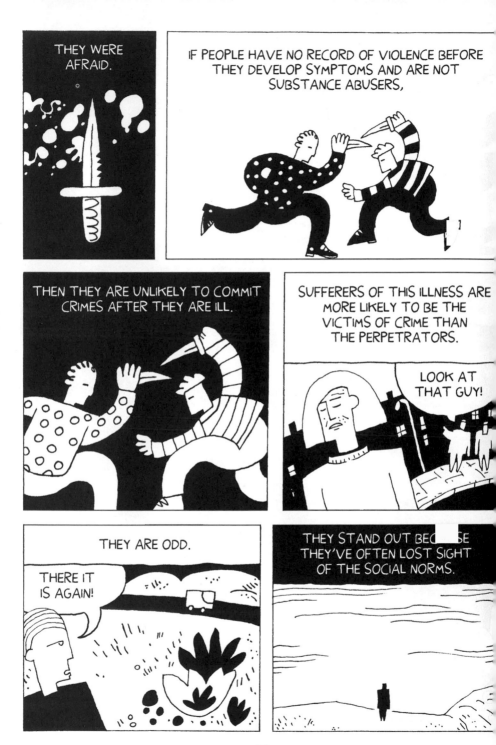

THEY ARE SUBJECT TO RIDICULE AND HOSTILITY.

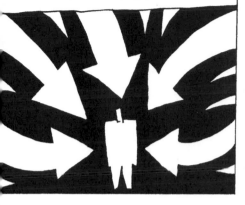

THEY ARE VULNERABLE.

THERE WAS A PARTICULAR PATIENT I REMEMBER.

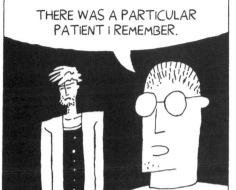

A MAN IN HIS FIFTIES, WHO WAS HALF-STARVED ON ADMISSION TO THE WARD.

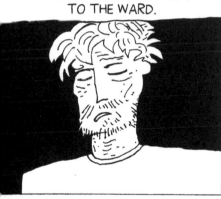

ORIGINALLY A PATIENT ON ONE OF THE OLD LONG STAY WARDS, HE'D BEEN MOVED OUT INTO THE COMMUNITY SOME YEARS BEFORE.

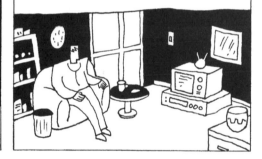

WHEN SOCIAL SERVICES CHECKED UP ON THIS MAN, THEY FOUND HIM LIVING IN SQUALOR.

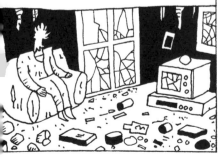

LOCAL YOUTHS HAD INSERTED THEMSELVES INTO HIS LIFE AND HOME,

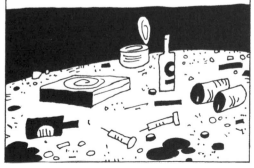

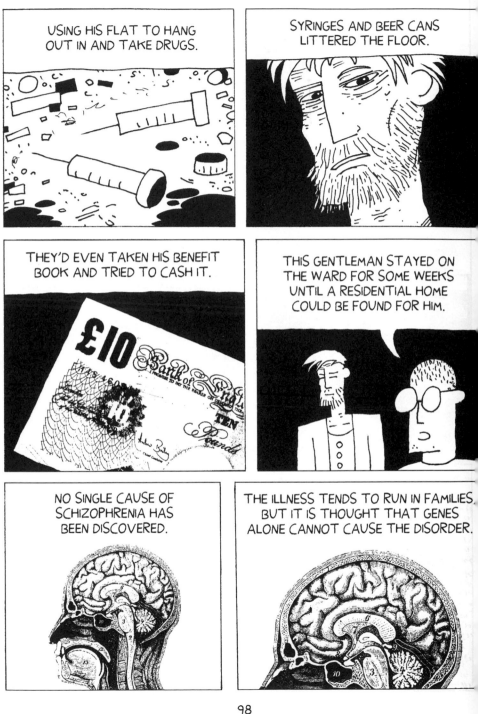

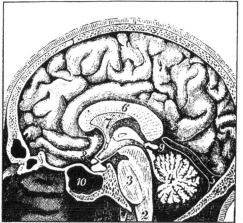

INTERACTION BETWEEN GENES AND THE ENVIRONMENT IS THOUGHT TO BE NECESSARY FOR SCHIZOPHRENIA TO DEVELOP.

MANY ENVIRONMENTAL FACTORS HAVE BEEN SUGGESTED AS RISK FACTORS.

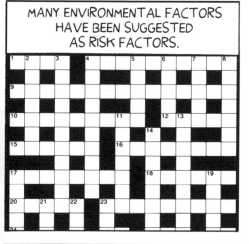

EXPOSURE TO VIRUSES OR MALNUTRITION IN THE WOMB,

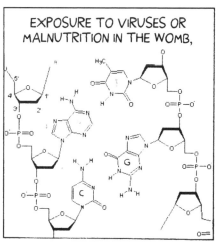

SUBTLE BRAIN DAMAGE AT BIRTH,

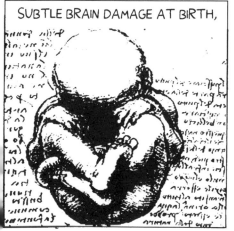

SOCIAL FACTORS SUCH AS STRESSFUL ENVIRONMENTAL CONDITIONS.

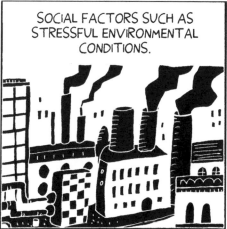

IN OTHER WORDS, ALMOST EVERYTHING IS IMPLICATED IN THE CAUSES OF SCHIZOPHRENIA,

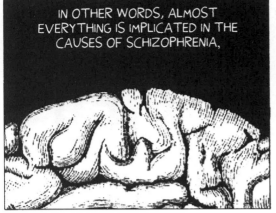

MAKING IT VERY DIFFICULT TO FOLLOW THE THREAD OF CAUSE AND EFFECT.

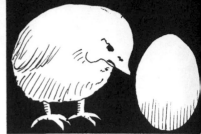

DO I HAVE TO TAKE ALL THESE?

YES, YOU DO.

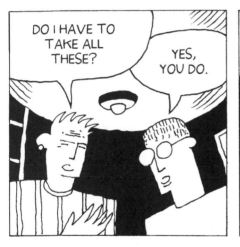

THE OLD ANTI-PSYCHOTIC MEDICATIONS, WHICH MANY STILL USE,

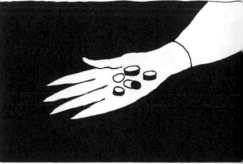

CAN CAUSE MUSCLE RIGIDITY, TREMORS, AND AGITATION, OBLIGING PEOPLE TO TAKE FURTHER DRUGS IN ORDER TO COUNTER THESE SIDE-EFFECTS.

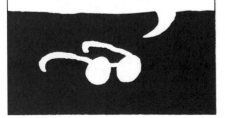

THE NEWER ANTI-PSYCHOTICS, WHICH WERE INTRODUCED IN THE 1990s, WORK WELL FOR THOSE WHOSE ILLNESS WAS PREVIOUSLY TREATMENT RESISTANT.

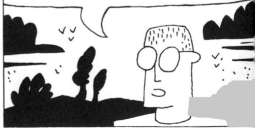

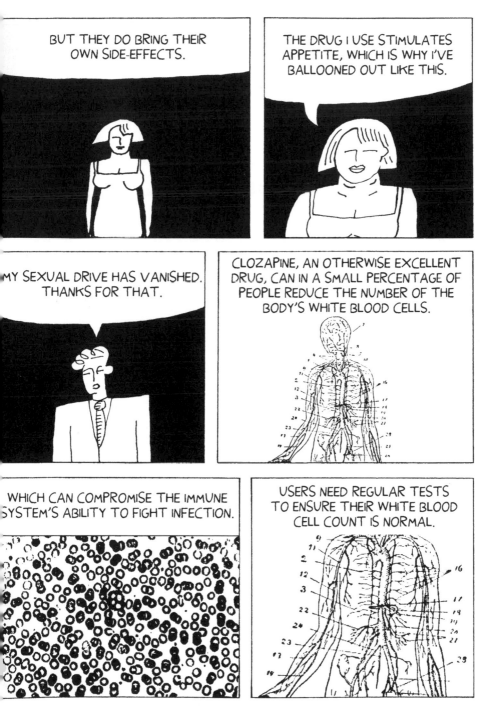

EVEN WITH THESE SIDE-EFFECTS, PEOPLE WHO SUFFER SEVERE SCHIZOPHRENIA ARE STILL FAR BETTER OFF WITH MEDICATION THAN IF THEY'D BEEN LEFT UNTREATED.

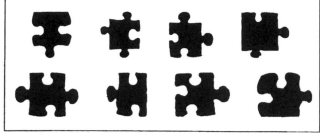

IN THE PAST, THEY'D BE CONSUMED BY MADNESS, OR FROZEN IN A STATE OF CATATONIA.

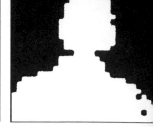

NOW THERE'S A BETTER CHANCE OF A NORMAL LIFE.

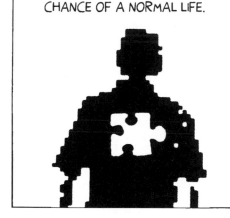

THE PUZZLE OF BRAIN ILLNESS IS BETTER UNDERSTOOD EVERY YEAR.

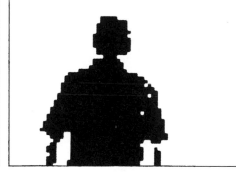

HOWEVER, THE GENERAL POPULATION NEEDS TO BE MORE UNDERSTANDING OF THOSE WHO SUFFER MENTAL ILLNESS.

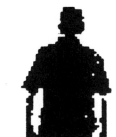

OUR LIVES ARE DIFFICULT ENOUGH AS IT IS.

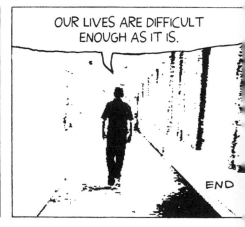

END

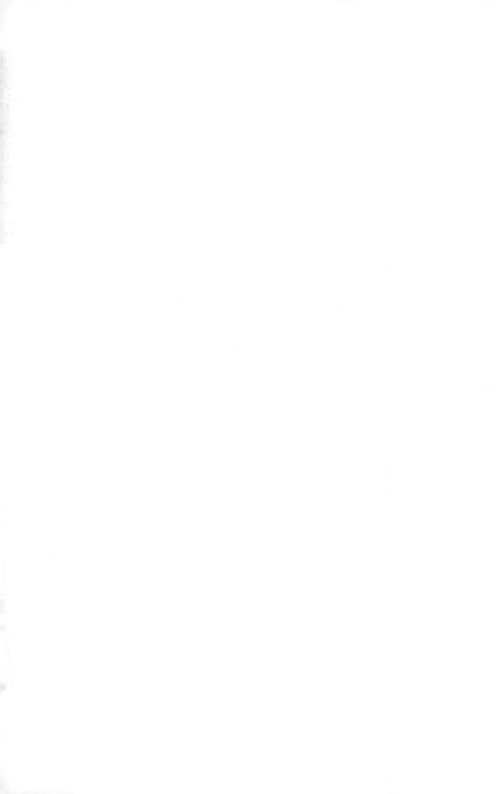

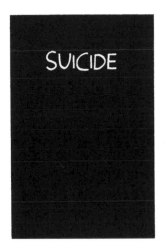

SUICIDE

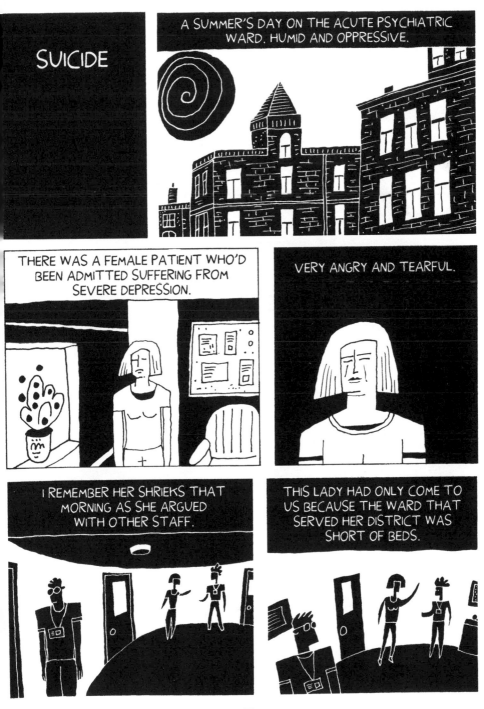

SUICIDE

A SUMMER'S DAY ON THE ACUTE PSYCHIATRIC WARD. HUMID AND OPPRESSIVE.

THERE WAS A FEMALE PATIENT WHO'D BEEN ADMITTED SUFFERING FROM SEVERE DEPRESSION.

VERY ANGRY AND TEARFUL.

I REMEMBER HER SHRIEKS THAT MORNING AS SHE ARGUED WITH OTHER STAFF.

THIS LADY HAD ONLY COME TO US BECAUSE THE WARD THAT SERVED HER DISTRICT WAS SHORT OF BEDS.

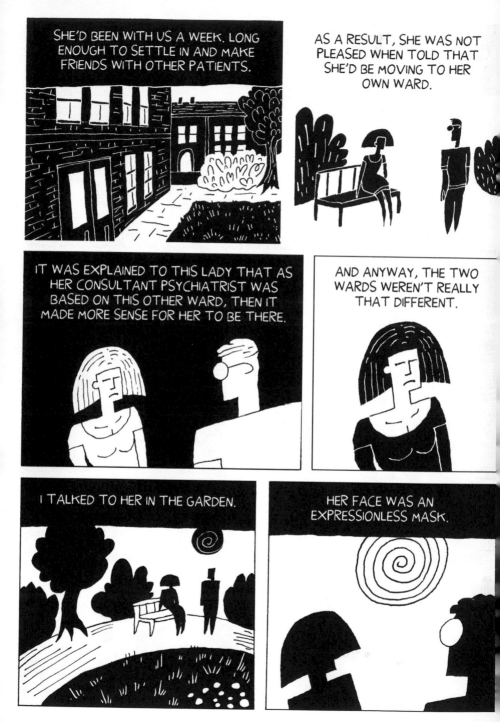

SHE'D BEEN WITH US A WEEK. LONG ENOUGH TO SETTLE IN AND MAKE FRIENDS WITH OTHER PATIENTS.

AS A RESULT, SHE WAS NOT PLEASED WHEN TOLD THAT SHE'D BE MOVING TO HER OWN WARD.

IT WAS EXPLAINED TO THIS LADY THAT AS HER CONSULTANT PSYCHIATRIST WAS BASED ON THIS OTHER WARD, THEN IT MADE MORE SENSE FOR HER TO BE THERE.

AND ANYWAY, THE TWO WARDS WEREN'T REALLY THAT DIFFERENT.

I TALKED TO HER IN THE GARDEN.

HER FACE WAS AN EXPRESSIONLESS MASK.

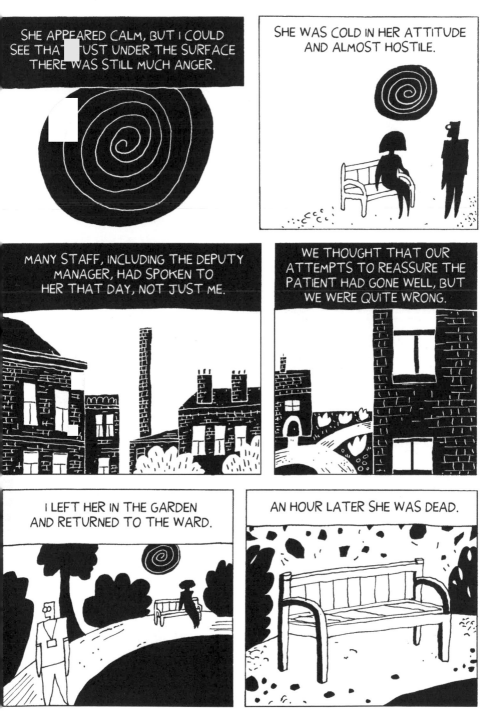

SHE APPEARED CALM, BUT I COULD SEE THAT JUST UNDER THE SURFACE THERE WAS STILL MUCH ANGER.

SHE WAS COLD IN HER ATTITUDE AND ALMOST HOSTILE.

MANY STAFF, INCLUDING THE DEPUTY MANAGER, HAD SPOKEN TO HER THAT DAY, NOT JUST ME.

WE THOUGHT THAT OUR ATTEMPTS TO REASSURE THE PATIENT HAD GONE WELL, BUT WE WERE QUITE WRONG.

I LEFT HER IN THE GARDEN AND RETURNED TO THE WARD.

AN HOUR LATER SHE WAS DEAD.

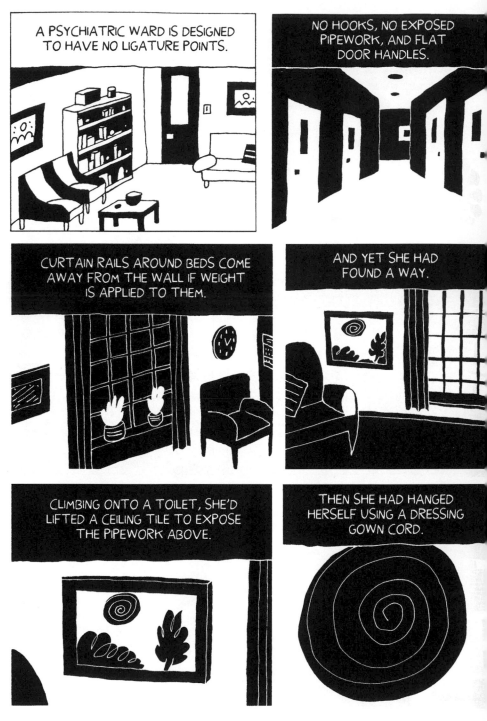

I REMEMBER THE SCREAMS OF THE YOUNG MEMBER OF STAFF WHO FOUND THE WOMAN.

THEY TRIED TO HOLD THE PATIENT UP IN ORDER TO RELIEVE THE PRESSURE ON HER AIRWAYS

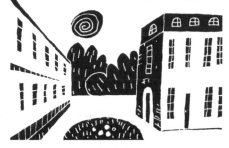

WHILE ATTEMPTING TO UNTIE THE CORD FROM THE PIPE.

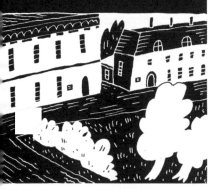

I SCRAMBLED TO THE OFFICE IN A SEARCH FOR SCISSORS.

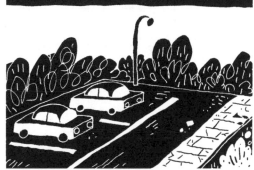

EVEN AFTER SHE WAS CUT DOWN THE NOOSE REMAINED TIGHT AROUND HER THROAT.

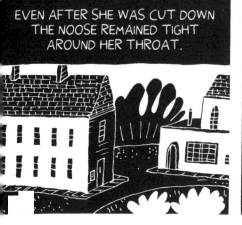

ITS GRIP CRUSHING HER WINDPIPE.

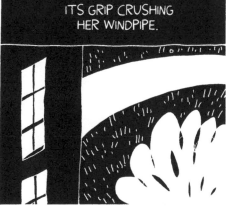

111

THEY COULD NOT SAVE HER.

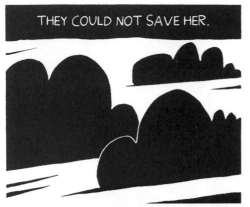

SHE DIED, LEAVING A YOUNG FAMILY BEHIND.

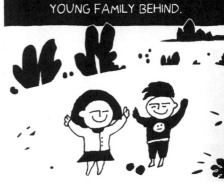

THE PATIENT HAD GIVEN US NO INDICATION THAT SHE WAS SUICIDAL.

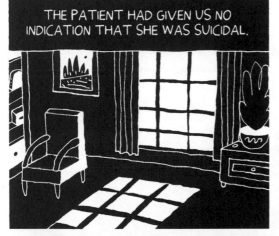

NOT A HINT OF WHAT SHE HAD PLANNED WAS PICKED UP BY STAFF.

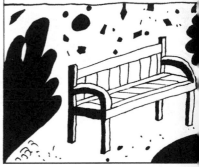

HER ANGER AND IMPASSIVITY HAD SUCCESSFULLY MASKED HER TRUE THOUGHTS.

SHE GAVE US NO CLUE BECAUSE SHE DIDN'T WANT TO BE SAVED.

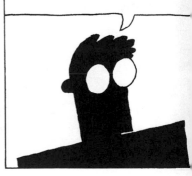

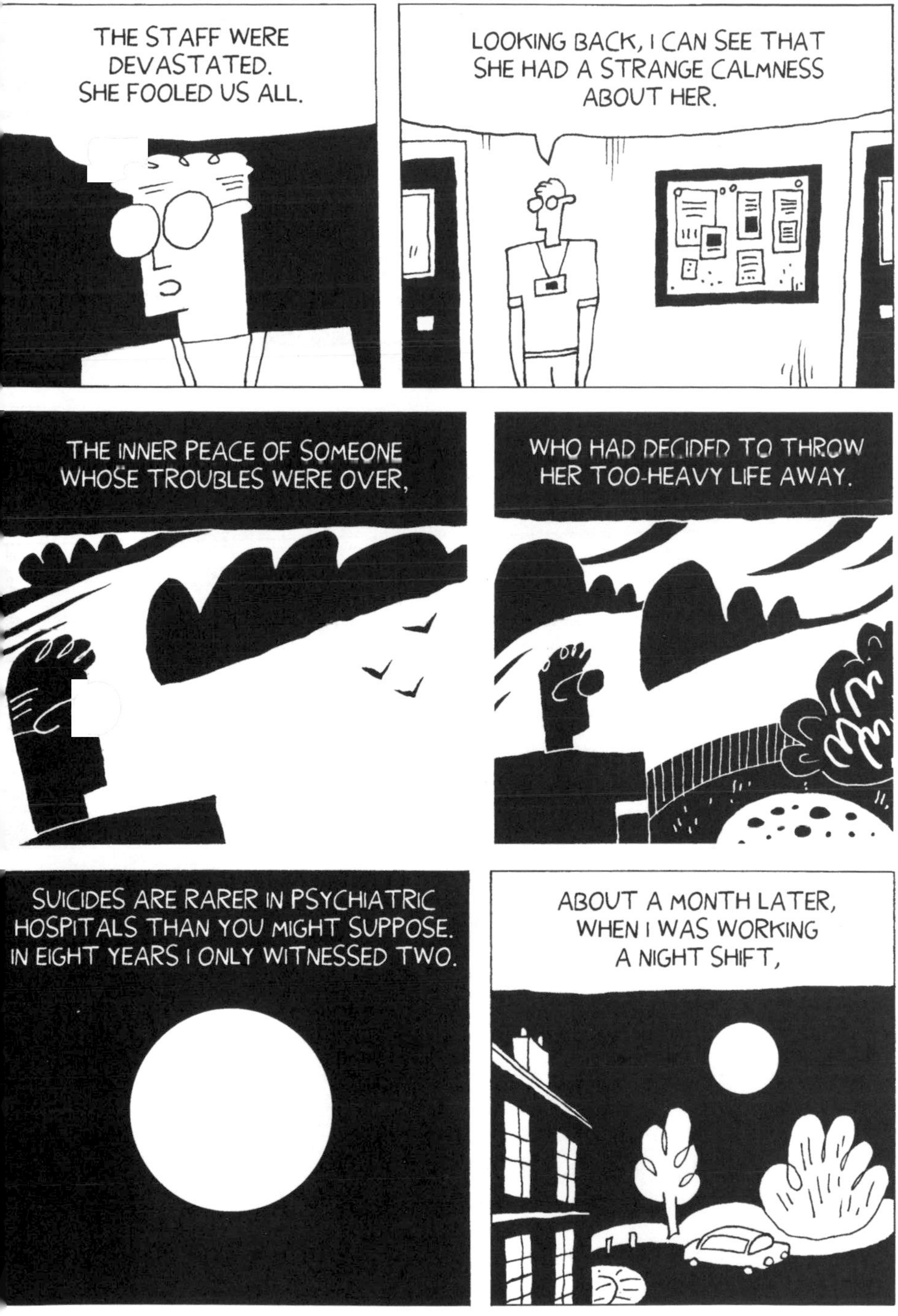

THE STAFF WERE DEVASTATED. SHE FOOLED US ALL.

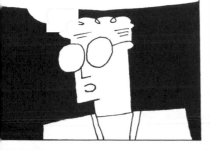

LOOKING BACK, I CAN SEE THAT SHE HAD A STRANGE CALMNESS ABOUT HER.

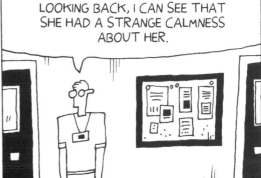

THE INNER PEACE OF SOMEONE WHOSE TROUBLES WERE OVER,

WHO HAD DECIDED TO THROW HER TOO-HEAVY LIFE AWAY.

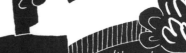

SUICIDES ARE RARER IN PSYCHIATRIC HOSPITALS THAN YOU MIGHT SUPPOSE. IN EIGHT YEARS I ONLY WITNESSED TWO.

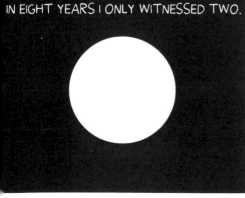

ABOUT A MONTH LATER, WHEN I WAS WORKING A NIGHT SHIFT,

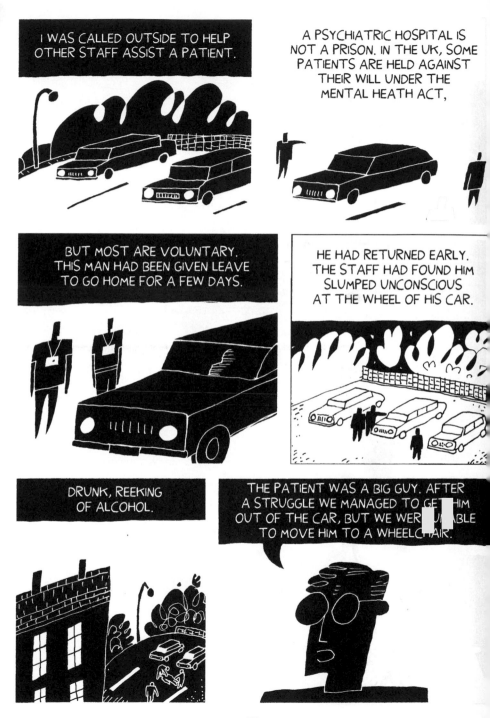

I WAS CALLED OUTSIDE TO HELP OTHER STAFF ASSIST A PATIENT.

A PSYCHIATRIC HOSPITAL IS NOT A PRISON. IN THE UK, SOME PATIENTS ARE HELD AGAINST THEIR WILL UNDER THE MENTAL HEATH ACT,

BUT MOST ARE VOLUNTARY. THIS MAN HAD BEEN GIVEN LEAVE TO GO HOME FOR A FEW DAYS.

HE HAD RETURNED EARLY. THE STAFF HAD FOUND HIM SLUMPED UNCONSCIOUS AT THE WHEEL OF HIS CAR.

DRUNK, REEKING OF ALCOHOL.

THE PATIENT WAS A BIG GUY. AFTER A STRUGGLE WE MANAGED TO GET HIM OUT OF THE CAR, BUT WE WERE UNABLE TO MOVE HIM TO A WHEELCHAIR.

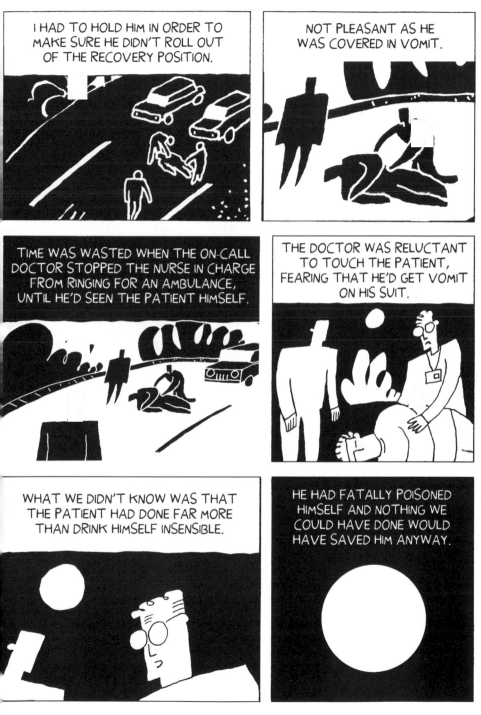

115

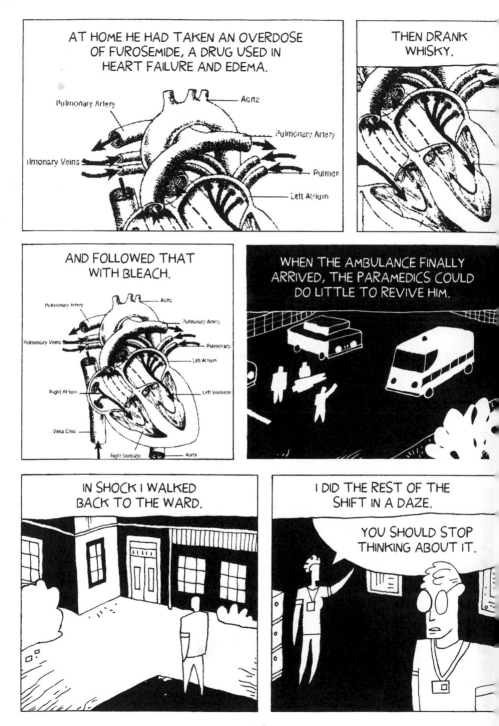

AT HOME HE HAD TAKEN AN OVERDOSE OF FUROSEMIDE, A DRUG USED IN HEART FAILURE AND EDEMA.

THEN DRANK WHISKY.

AND FOLLOWED THAT WITH BLEACH.

WHEN THE AMBULANCE FINALLY ARRIVED, THE PARAMEDICS COULD DO LITTLE TO REVIVE HIM.

IN SHOCK I WALKED BACK TO THE WARD.

I DID THE REST OF THE SHIFT IN A DAZE.

YOU SHOULD STOP THINKING ABOUT IT.

116

WHY HAD HE DONE SUCH A THING TO HIMSELF?

WHAT WAS HIS MOTIVATION IN DRIVING BACK TO THE HOSPITAL? DID HE HOPE TO BE FOUND?

I FELT AN AWFUL GUILT. WOULD THE PATIENT STILL BE ALIVE IF WE'D DONE MORE AND REACTED SOONER?

WOULD IT HAVE MADE ANY DIFFERENCE IF THE PARAMEDICS HAD ARRIVED EARLIER?

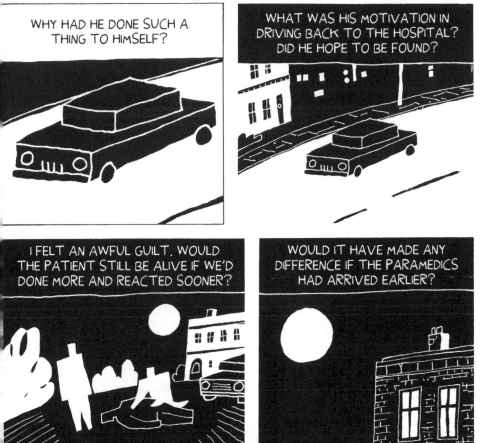

PROBABLY NOT, BUT I COULD NEVER BE SURE, AND THIS FACT HAUNTED ME FOR YEARS.

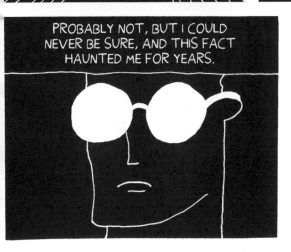

THE EFFECTS OF SUICIDE RIPPLE OUTWARD.

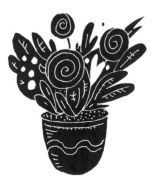

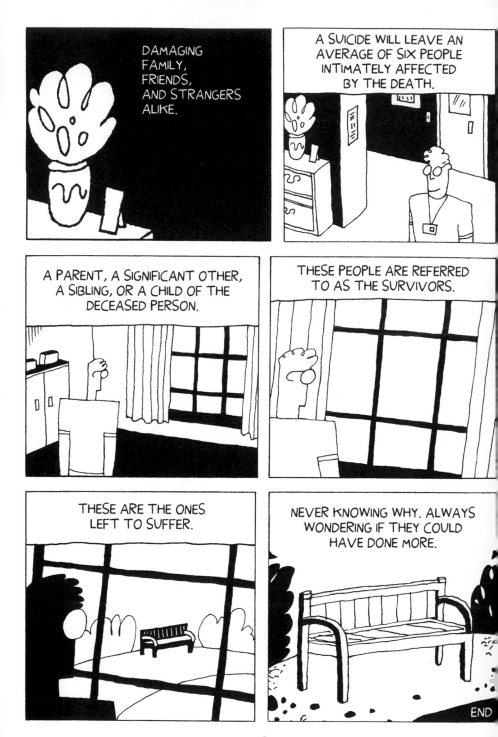

DAMAGING FAMILY, FRIENDS, AND STRANGERS ALIKE.

A SUICIDE WILL LEAVE AN AVERAGE OF SIX PEOPLE INTIMATELY AFFECTED BY THE DEATH.

A PARENT, A SIGNIFICANT OTHER, A SIBLING, OR A CHILD OF THE DECEASED PERSON.

THESE PEOPLE ARE REFERRED TO AS THE SURVIVORS.

THESE ARE THE ONES LEFT TO SUFFER.

NEVER KNOWING WHY. ALWAYS WONDERING IF THEY COULD HAVE DONE MORE.

END

HOW I LIVED AGAIN

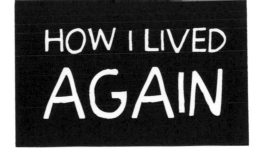

HOW I LIVED AGAIN

MY LIFE DURING THE WRITING OF THIS BOOK HAS BEEN SOMETHING OF A STRUGGLE.

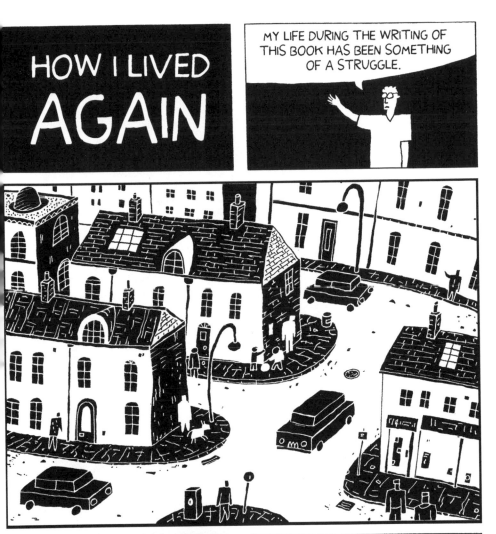

BETWEEN THE CHAPTER ON ANTI-SOCIAL PERSONALITY DISORDER

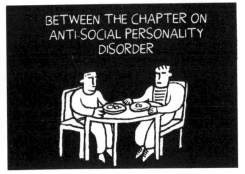

AND THE CHAPTER ON FAMOUS PEOPLE WHO HAVE SUFFERED A MENTAL ILLNESS,

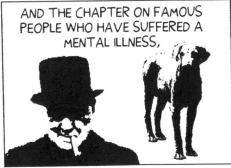

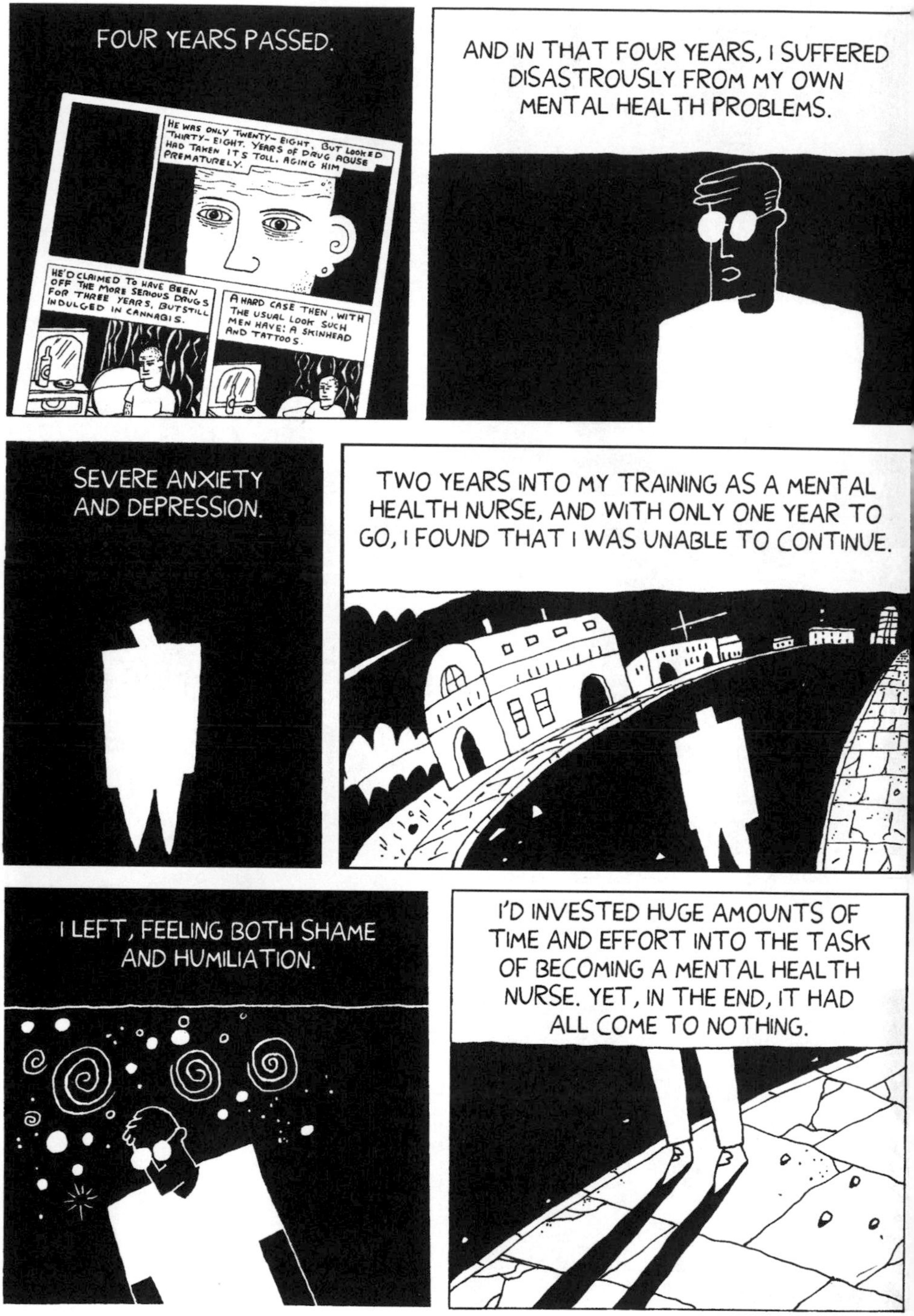
FOUR YEARS PASSED.
HE WAS ONLY TWENTY-EIGHT, BUT LOOKED THIRTY-EIGHT. YEARS OF DRUG ABUSE HAD TAKEN ITS TOLL, AGING HIM PREMATURELY.
HE'D CLAIMED TO HAVE BEEN OFF THE MORE SERIOUS DRUGS FOR THREE YEARS, BUT STILL INDULGED IN CANNABIS.
A HARD CASE THEN, WITH THE USUAL LOOK SUCH MEN HAVE: A SKINHEAD AND TATTOOS.
AND IN THAT FOUR YEARS, I SUFFERED DISASTROUSLY FROM MY OWN MENTAL HEALTH PROBLEMS.
SEVERE ANXIETY AND DEPRESSION.
TWO YEARS INTO MY TRAINING AS A MENTAL HEALTH NURSE, AND WITH ONLY ONE YEAR TO GO, I FOUND THAT I WAS UNABLE TO CONTINUE.
I LEFT, FEELING BOTH SHAME AND HUMILIATION.
I'D INVESTED HUGE AMOUNTS OF TIME AND EFFORT INTO THE TASK OF BECOMING A MENTAL HEALTH NURSE. YET, IN THE END, IT HAD ALL COME TO NOTHING.

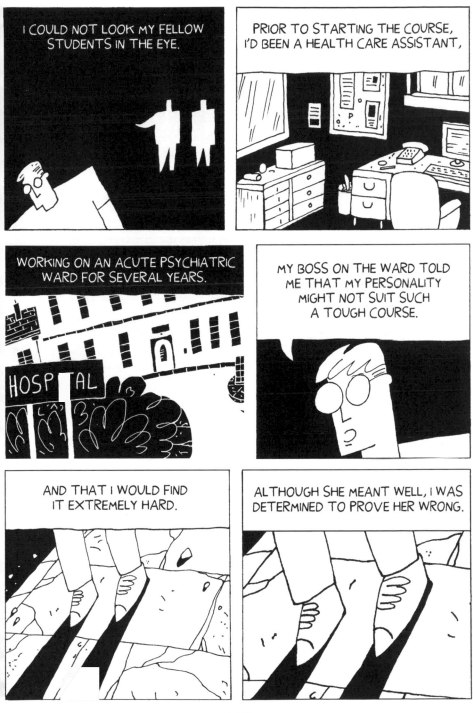

I COULD NOT LOOK MY FELLOW STUDENTS IN THE EYE.

PRIOR TO STARTING THE COURSE, I'D BEEN A HEALTH CARE ASSISTANT,

WORKING ON AN ACUTE PSYCHIATRIC WARD FOR SEVERAL YEARS.

HOSPITAL

MY BOSS ON THE WARD TOLD ME THAT MY PERSONALITY MIGHT NOT SUIT SUCH A TOUGH COURSE.

AND THAT I WOULD FIND IT EXTREMELY HARD.

ALTHOUGH SHE MEANT WELL, I WAS DETERMINED TO PROVE HER WRONG.

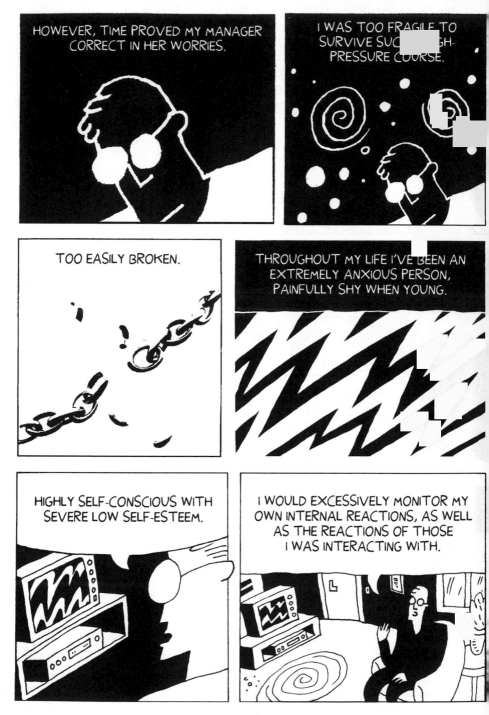

HOWEVER, TIME PROVED MY MANAGER CORRECT IN HER WORRIES.

I WAS TOO FRAGILE TO SURVIVE SUC? ??GH- PRESSURE COURSE.

TOO EASILY BROKEN.

THROUGHOUT MY LIFE I'VE BEEN AN EXTREMELY ANXIOUS PERSON, PAINFULLY SHY WHEN YOUNG.

HIGHLY SELF-CONSCIOUS WITH SEVERE LOW SELF-ESTEEM.

I WOULD EXCESSIVELY MONITOR MY OWN INTERNAL REACTIONS, AS WELL AS THE REACTIONS OF THOSE I WAS INTERACTING WITH.

THIS CREATED AN EXTREME TENSION WITHIN MYSELF. I WAS SO PREOCCUPIED WITH MONITORING MYSELF AND OTHERS

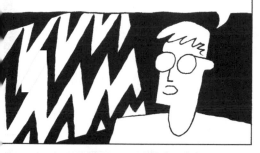

THAT I FOUND IT DIFFICULT TO PRODUCE FLUENT SPEECH.

UH!

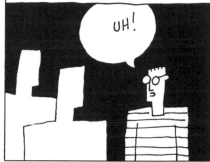

IT WAS FAR EASIER FOR ME TO REMAIN SILENT IN SOCIAL SITUATIONS.

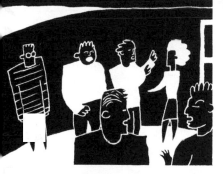

THIS WAS MORE THAN JUST SHYNESS. IT WAS A SOCIAL ANXIETY DISORDER WITH DEEP CONSEQUENCES.

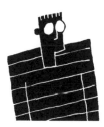
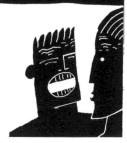

I EXPERIENCED A CONSTANT FEELING OF TENSION AND FEAR.

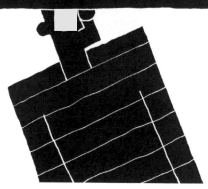

I HAD A STRONG BELIEF THAT I WAS SOCIALLY INEPT AND INFERIOR TO OTHERS.

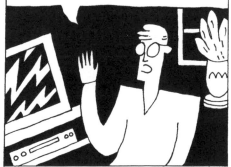

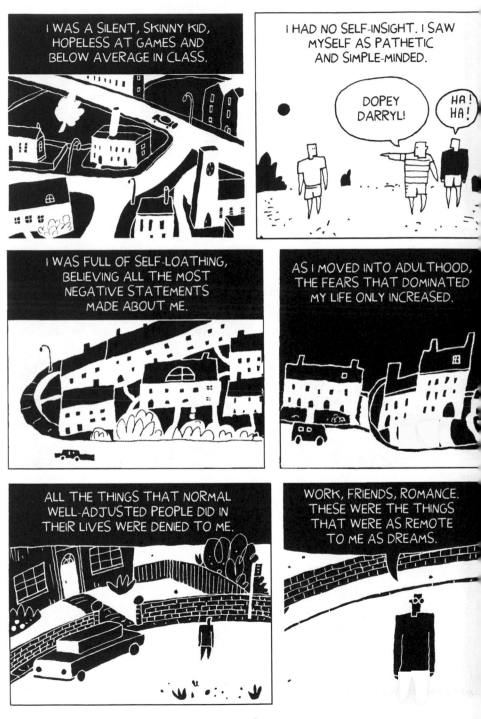

128

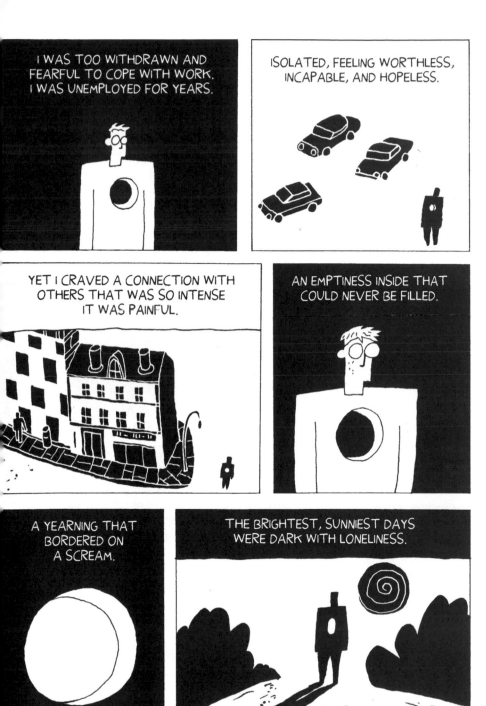

LIFE IMPROVED WITH
GLACIAL SLOWNESS.

I GRADUALLY DEVELOPED A SMALL
AMOUNT OF SELF-WORTH
THROUGH ARTISTIC TALENT.

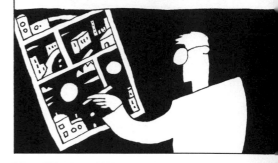

I WAS CREATIVE AND
IMAGINATIVE.

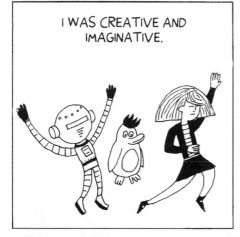

PARTICULARLY GOOD AT DRAWING
URBAN LANDSCAPES, STREETS,
TOWNS, AND CITIES.

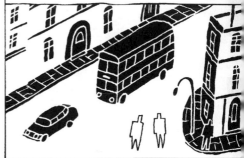

I CULTIVATED FRIENDSHIPS WITH
OTHER TALENTED PEOPLE.

I BEGAN TO SEE MYSELF AS
PART OF A COMMUNITY OF
CARTOONISTS AND
ILLUSTRATORS.

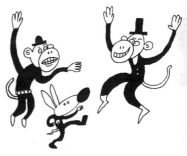

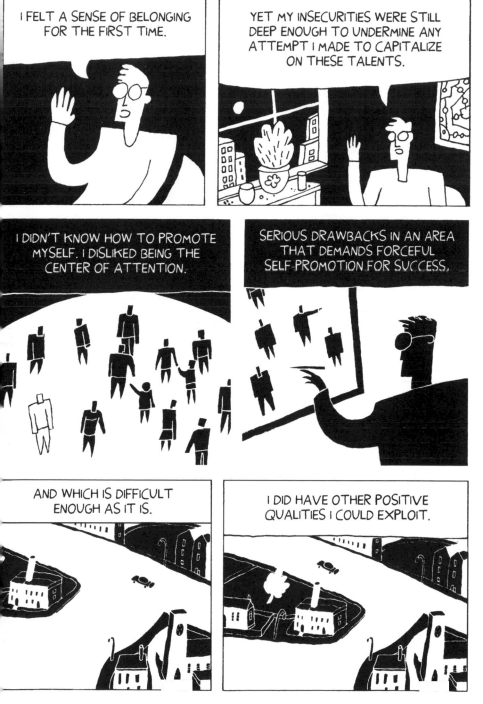

PERHAPS BECAUSE I WAS SO IMAGINATIVE, I FOUND IT EASY TO PLACE MYSELF IN ANOTHER'S SHOES.

I WAS NATURALLY KIND AND HAD A GREAT DEAL OF PATIENCE.

MY INTEREST IN MENTAL HEALTH ISSUES, STEMMING FROM AN ATTEMPT TO UNDERSTAND MY OWN PROBLEMS,

LED ME INTO MENTAL HEALTH WORK.

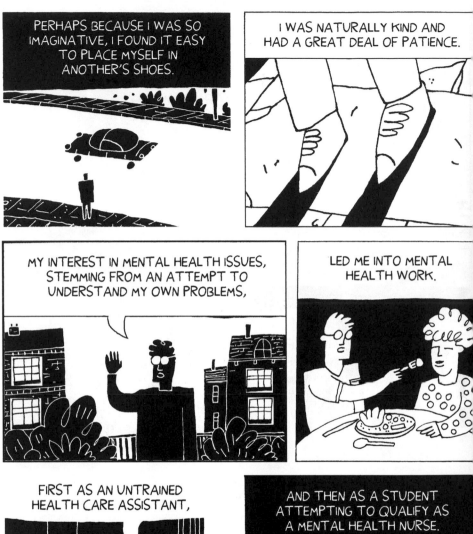

FIRST AS AN UNTRAINED HEALTH CARE ASSISTANT,

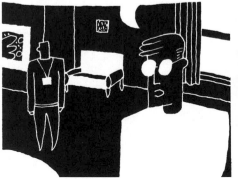

AND THEN AS A STUDENT ATTEMPTING TO QUALIFY AS A MENTAL HEALTH NURSE.

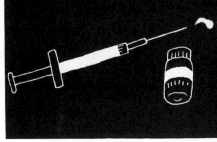

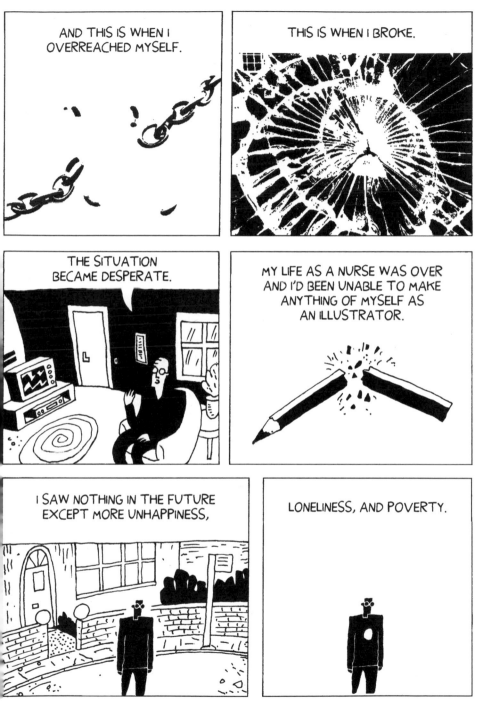

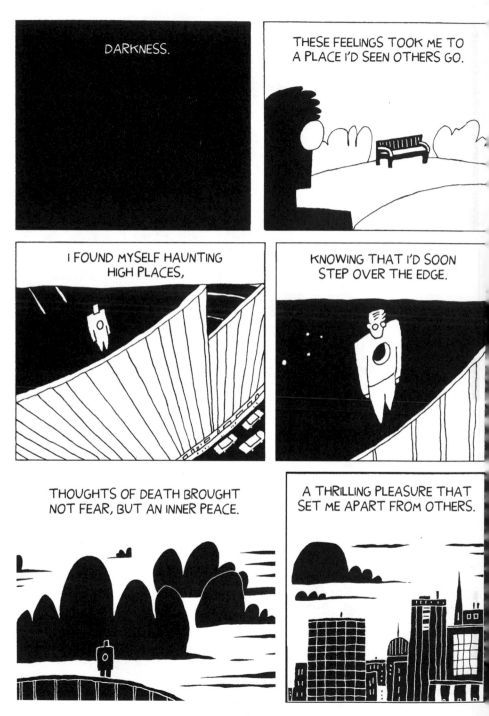

134

I RAN UP HUGE DEBTS, THINKING THAT IT DIDN'T MATTER ANYWAY, AS I WOULDN'T BE AROUND TO HAVE TO PAY THEM OFF.

GRADUALLY, DESPITE MYSELF, I RETURNED TO THE WORLD OF THE LIVING.

TWO THINGS CHANGED MY LIFE: PROZAC AND THE INTERNET.

PROZAC HELPED LIFT MY LOW MOOD.

WHILE THE INTERNET HELPED ME PROMOTE MYSELF AS AN ARTIST.

I BEGAN TO GET A REGULAR AUDIENCE THROUGH VARIOUS ONLINE SOCIAL NETWORKS.

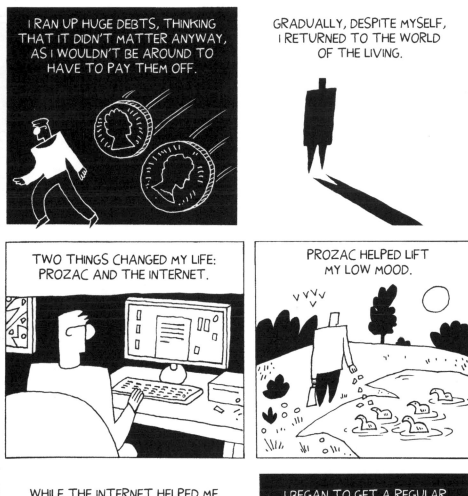

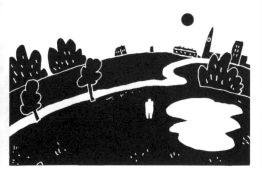

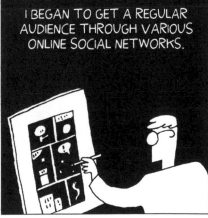

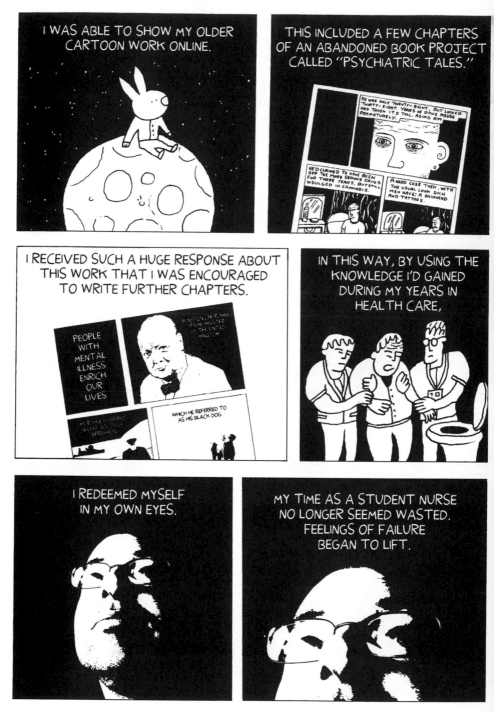

I WAS ABLE TO SHOW MY OLDER CARTOON WORK ONLINE.

THIS INCLUDED A FEW CHAPTERS OF AN ABANDONED BOOK PROJECT CALLED "PSYCHIATRIC TALES."

I RECEIVED SUCH A HUGE RESPONSE ABOUT THIS WORK THAT I WAS ENCOURAGED TO WRITE FURTHER CHAPTERS.

IN THIS WAY, BY USING THE KNOWLEDGE I'D GAINED DURING MY YEARS IN HEALTH CARE,

I REDEEMED MYSELF IN MY OWN EYES.

MY TIME AS A STUDENT NURSE NO LONGER SEEMED WASTED. FEELINGS OF FAILURE BEGAN TO LIFT.

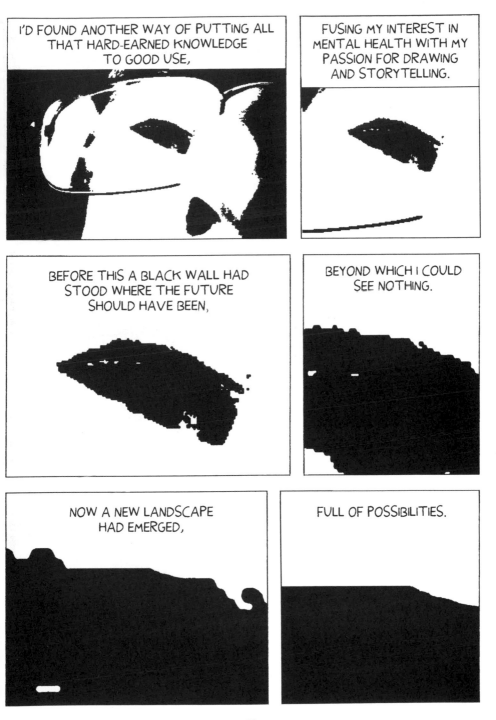

I'D FOUND ANOTHER WAY OF PUTTING ALL THAT HARD-EARNED KNOWLEDGE TO GOOD USE,

FUSING MY INTEREST IN MENTAL HEALTH WITH MY PASSION FOR DRAWING AND STORYTELLING.

BEFORE THIS A BLACK WALL HAD STOOD WHERE THE FUTURE SHOULD HAVE BEEN,

BEYOND WHICH I COULD SEE NOTHING.

NOW A NEW LANDSCAPE HAD EMERGED,

FULL OF POSSIBILITIES.

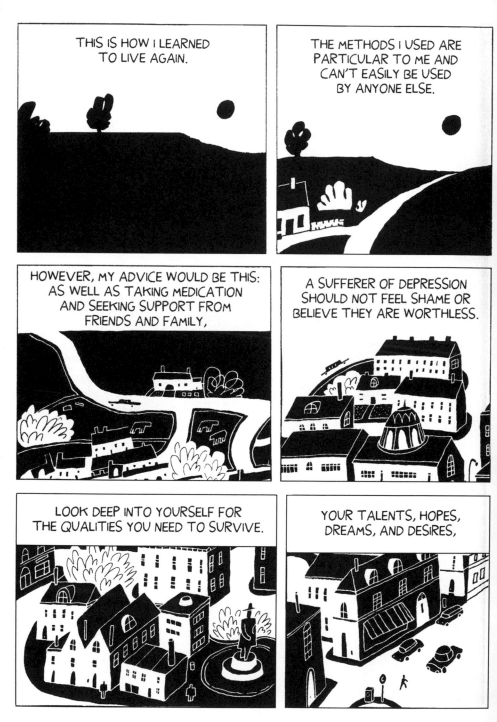

138

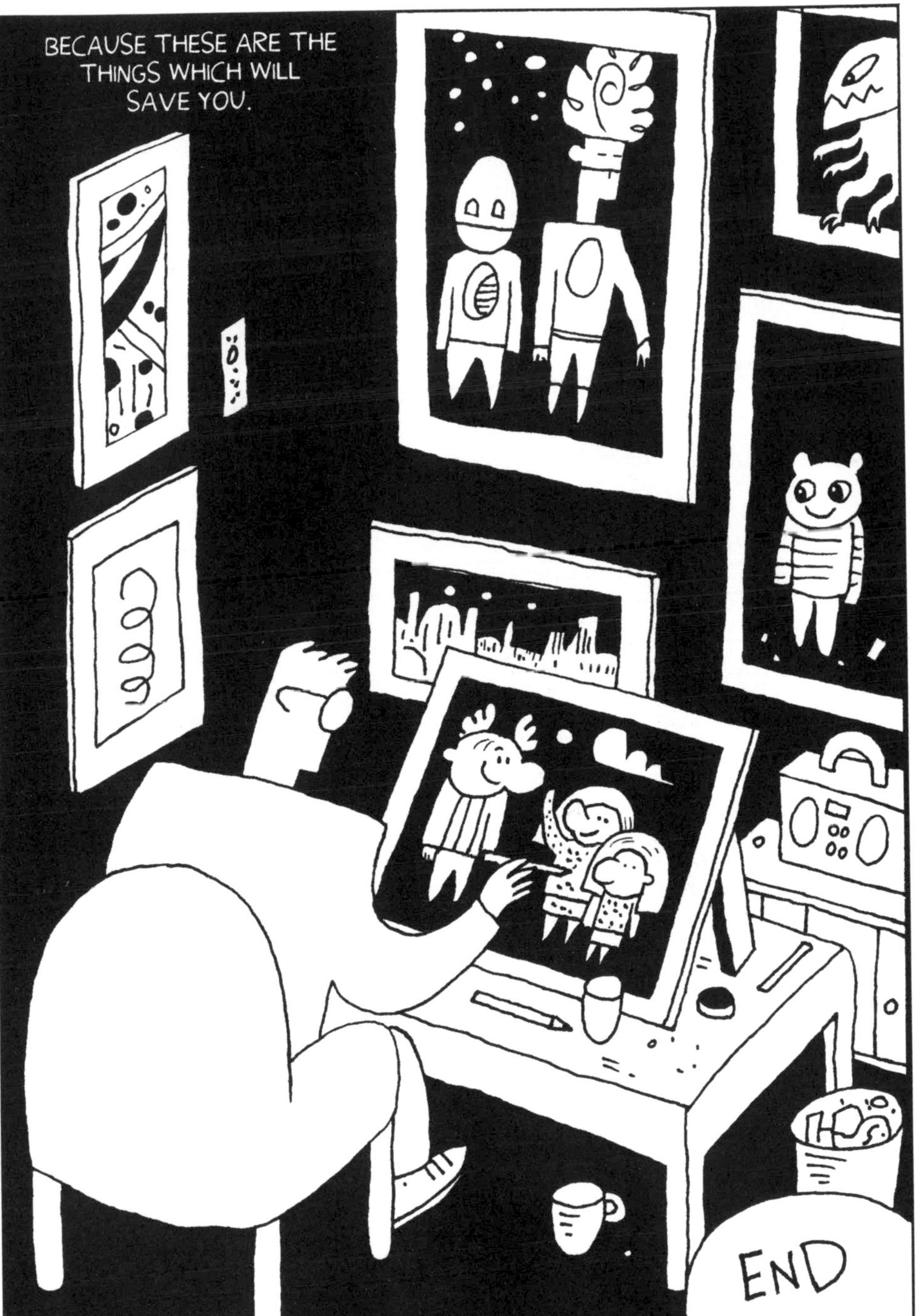
BECAUSE THESE ARE THE THINGS WHICH WILL SAVE YOU.
END

A NOTE ON THE AUTHOR

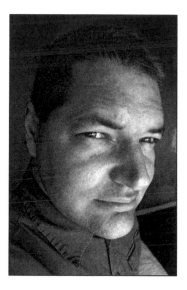

DARRYL CUNNINGHAM went to Leeds College of Art. He is a prolific cartoonist, sculptor, and photographer. His long stint working as a health care assistant on an acute psychiatric ward was the inspiration for this book. He is the creator of the Web comics "Super-Sam and John-of-the-Night" and "The Streets of San Diablo." He lives in Yorkshire, England.